TEACHING YOGA
&
MEDITATION
BEYOND
THE POSES

Cover & Graphic Design

Mattias Långström

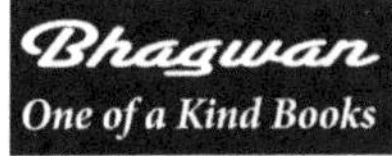

TEACHING YOGA
&
MEDITATION
BEYOND
THE POSES

ISBN 9789198839333

✳✳✳

Publisher **BHAGWAN 2023**

THE BOOK

Teaching Yoga and Meditation Beyond the Poses – An unique and practical workbook for aspiring yoga teachers that want to teach yoga and meditation beyond the poses.

Teaching Yoga and Meditation Beyond the Poses is a new edition of the popular Yoga Bible, with clearer typography, a smarter format and at a lower price. The book is a unique and essential resource for new and experienced teachers as well as a guide for all yoga students interested in refining their skills and knowledge. Teaching Yoga and Meditation is also ideal for use as a core textbook in yoga teacher training programs.

The book covers fundamental topics of yoga philosophy and history, including a historical presentation of classical yoga literature: Yoga Sutras of Patanjali, Bhagavad Gita, etc. Each of the seven major styles of yoga is described, from Hatha yoga, Raja yoga, Tantra yoga, Bhakti yoga, and Kundalini yoga to knowledge about the chakras, Ayurveda and magic mantras and yantras. The book provides extensive support and tools for teaching integrated and classical yoga (asanas), breathing techniques (pranayama), deep relaxation (Yoga Nidra) and meditation (Ajapa Japa). The book is divided into eight modules with associated knowledge tests and complete yoga and meditation classes.

Shreyananda Natha is a bestselling author of yoga books.

REVIEW 5 STAR

"Really good fact/study book on yoga! Have just had time to go through the whole book and I think it is super good. Now I am a Kundalini yoga teacher but am thinking of including it in my teaching for future yoga teachers. If all teacher training could follow the 8 modules, we would have very knowledgeable yoga teachers. A big plus is that it is so wide. From Hatha yoga to Kundalini yoga, meditation, chakras and mantra magic. Good that it also had a module about Ayurveda. Recommended!" – **Benny Rosen YOGA TEACHER**

Namasté

I want to thank the teachers and students I have had over the years who have made my journey with yoga so interesting. Thank you for all the inspiration you have given me and for making this book possible. The yoga masters who no longer live among us, live on with every new person who immerses themselves in the yoga tradition.

Sri Swami Sivananda, Sri Swami Satyananda, Sri Tirumalai Krishnamacharya, Sri Swami Vishnudevananda, Sri K. Pattabhi Jois, Osho, Swami Nirdosha, Swami Omananda, Swami Janakananda, Ole Schmidt, Turiya, Maryam Abrishami and Sanna Kuittinen.

Everyone has searched for answers to what they perceived through an activated ajna chakra. In yoga, they have learned the principles behind the universe, the collective consciousness, and the creative power, Kundalini Shakti. The duality behind everything, both what we see and what we do not see. Together we help to pass on the previous secret knowledge, about our gunas, nadis, and chakras, to anyone who wants to be seen.

THE AUTHOR

Shreyananda Natha is the author of over twelve titles on yoga. Among other things, he has written the most comprehensive books on yoga in Swedish – Everything About Yoga and the study book The Yoga Bible. He is also a certified yoga and meditation teacher according to EYTF's international guidelines and has undergone multi-year yoga teacher training under the leadership of Swami Omananda at Satyananda Ashram. Shreyananda Natha holds the highest initiation in the Tantric Natha Order. He travels frequently to Asia and India to improve himself, and to gain knowledge and inspiration. He has immersed himself in tantric rituals and is known for his extensive knowledge of yoga, deep relaxation, and meditation.

"There is no authority that can say what yoga is. When you give yourself fully and completely and experience yoga without limitations or doubts, when you become one with the true experience in yourself, the real encounter with yoga arises. Only then do you understand what yoga is – for you. You are no longer limited by ornament, shyness and artificial thought patterns that lie as a filter between you and the transformation. Yoga is a cultural-historical wealth that is still passed on from teacher to student and helps man to find his way back to his true nature. It opens us up and attracts awareness. It strengthens our self-esteem, and our entire personal spectrum of possibilities suddenly becomes visible to us. Yoga is not difficult. You do not have to be vegan or able to stand on your head. You just need to practice your yoga regularly and the rest will come by itself."

With all the love from the universe – Aum Shanti

Shreyananda Natha.

INDEX

PREFACE

Teaching Yoga and Meditation Beyond the Poses – An unique and practical workbook for aspiring yoga teachers that want to teach yoga and meditation beyond the poses.

The book covers fundamental topics of yoga philosophy and history, including a historical presentation of classical yoga literature: Yoga Sutras of Patanjali, Bhagavad Gita, etc. Each of the seven major styles of yoga is described, from Hatha yoga, Raja yoga, Tantra yoga, Bhakti yoga, and Kundalini yoga to knowledge about the chakras, Ayurveda and magic mantras and yantras. The book provides extensive support and tools for teaching integrated and classical yoga (asanas), breathing techniques (pranayama), deep relaxation (Yoga Nidra) and meditation (Ajapa Japa). The book is divided into eight modules with associated knowledge tests and complete yoga and meditation classes.

As a complement to Teaching Yoga and Meditation Beyond the Poses, the book Best Book for yoga lovers – 3 books in one, comprising three classic yoga books (Hatha Yoga Pradipika, Patanjali Yoga Sutras and Kundalini Yoga) is recommended.

Module 1. The origin and history of yoga as well as orientation in yoga and the esoteric evolution of yoga and tantra through the 36 tantric tattwas.

We study the history and origins of yoga and become acquainted with the theory behind Hatha yoga. We study the Ajna chakra and practice our exercises to cleanse, balance and activate the chakra. We start practicing in the role of yoga teacher with lesson no. 1 of 8.

Module 2. We study Hatha yoga from a practical perspective and immerse ourselves in the theory.

We study purification processes (shatkarma), the most important postures (asa-

na), breathing exercises (pranayama), postures (mudras), locks (bandhas) and get an orientation in the pranic (energy) body. We study the Mooladhara chakra and practice our exercises to cleanse, balance and activate the chakra. We continue to practice in the role of yoga teacher with lesson no. 2 of 8.

Module 3. Raja yoga, Patanjalis Yoga Sutra and meditation. We study the yoga philosophy and learn to lead yoga nidra and ajapa japa.

We study Raja yoga and yoga philosophy by reading the most important sutras from Patanjali's classic work, Yoga Sutra. We learn to lead the meditation ajapa japa and the deep relaxation yoga nidra, both from the tantric tradition. We study the Swadhisthana chakra and practice our exercises to cleanse, balance and activate the chakra. We continue to practice the role of yoga teacher with lesson no. 3 of 8.

Module 4. Kundalini yoga. We study the Kundalini Shakti and the chakra system and learn the principles behind awakening our latent powers.

We study Kundalini Shakti and her various names and immerse ourselves in the chakra system and its inherent forces and influence on our life potential. We are also beginning to approach Kriya yoga. We study the Manipura chakra and practice our own exercises to cleanse, balance and activate the chakra. We continue to practice in the role of yoga teacher with lesson no. 4 of 8.

Module 5. Karma, Bhakti and Jnana yoga. We study yoga from a Hindu perspective.

We study Karma, Bhakti and Jnana yoga and its context. We study the Anahata chakra and practice our exercises to cleanse, balance and activate the chakra. We continue to practice in the role of yoga teacher with lesson no. 5 of 8.

Module 6. Tantra and tattwa shuddhi. We study tantra and pancha tattwa – the five elements.

*We study tantra and the ancient technique of purifying the five elements –
tattwa shuddhi. We study the Vishuddhi chakra and practice our exercises to
cleanse, balance and activate the chakra. We continue to practice in the role of
yoga teacher with lesson no. 6 of 8.*

*Module 7. Ayurveda. We study vata, pitta, kapha and yoga's effect on the three
doshas as well as Ayurvedic treatments.*

*We study Ayurveda and our three doshas – vata, pitta and kapha - and how
they are affected by yoga and diet. We also familiarize ourselves with basic pulse
diagnostics. We read about Ayurvedic treatments such as pancha karma and the
importance of sesame oil. We study the Bindu visarga and practice our exercises
to cleanse, balance and activate chakras. We continue to practice in the role of
yoga teacher with lesson no.7 of 8.*

*Module 8. Esoteric yoga. We study some of the most secret and advanced yogic
techniques to awaken the hidden power that lies dormant within us.*

*We study some of the most advanced and secret techniques to awaken Kunda-
lini Shakti within us and become acquainted with the tantra of the right and
left paths. We read about secret chakras, magical mantras, Kriya yoga as well
as maithuna and sex magic. We study Sahasrara chakra and practice our own
exercises for an integrated chakra awakening. We continue to practice in the role
of yoga teacher with lesson no. 8 of 8.*

ADDITIONS TO THE BOOK

*There have been some things I have taken into account when deciding how to ex-
plain yoga in the book. According to tradition, the knowledge of yoga is handed
down from master to student. This largely oral tradition means that there may
be some differences in interpretation.*

*In India, there is also a culture of respecting different points of view. If you ask
a Hindu if he believes in Buddha, for example, he may answer that Buddha*

is great and an important god to believe in, as he is an incarnation of the god Krishna. It is very much a Western invention to exclude opinions. That something is right or wrong, that there is only one truth, is an uncompromising way of thinking which creates sects and suffocates the most important thing of all - our inner voice, our common sense.

One can argue endlessly about how many nadis there are in the body – is it about seventy-two thousand or about three hundred thousand, as well as how certain words should be spelled in Sanskrit. No one knows exactly, but everyone passes on their own inherited knowledge by tradition and therefore this book's knowledge is based on the truth that is most often considered prevalent at this time. When I lecture about yoga I say - in yoga some people think that ...

WHO SHOULD WE BELIEVE IN?

When you awaken the Ajna chakra and activate the pineal gland, your intuition will increase. You will be guided by an inner voice. Accept the knowledge in front of you, but always listen to the knowledge inside of you. Trust your intuition and let it grow, because it will show you the way. This is what will make you a great yoga master at some point in the future.

Many people try to take credit for yoga. Put their name before yoga knowledge and claim it as theirs. No authority can determine what yoga is. It is when you lie there and for the first time experience happiness in your innermost being – that it will suddenly dawn on you what yoga is. Just like the taste of a fruit, it must be experienced to be understood. Listen humbly to both the initiated and experienced, but never forget that we are all different. Yoga should expand and liberate you – make you grow. Yoga should make you more you.

To become a yogi – is to choose to improve oneself. To become the best version of yourself, regardless of your starting point in life. Yoga gives us the strength and belief to influence ourselves and our life situations.

The book is my initiation for you, in the yoga tradition. I pass on the knowledge that my yoga masters have given me and this does not have to be the only truth or the only correct interpretation. If you then like it, I would be incredibly grateful if you took the time to leave an honest review. One line or five doesn't matter, I'm grateful for all the support. It helps me when I'm trying to reach out with my books.

Thanks and good luck on your journey!

Shreyananda Natha.

MODULE 1

ORIGIN AND HISTORY OF YOGA AND ORIENTATION IN THE ESOTERIC EVOLUTION OF YOGA AND TANTRA THROUGH THE 36 TANTRA TATTWAS

We study the history and origins of yoga and become familiar with the theory behind Hatha yoga. We study the Ajna chakra and practice our exercises to cleanse, balance and activate the chakra. We start practicing in the role of yoga teacher with lesson no. 1 of 8.

Knowledge test: Answer the questions that relate to module 1. Practice lesson no. 1 with at least 1 participant and humbly accept feedback from them. Ask questions afterward – how was the pace, how did you keep to time, did you speak loudly enough and how well did you understand the exercises?

According to tradition, the knowledge of yoga is passed on from master to student in descending line. This largely oral tradition means that there may be some differences in interpretation.

WHAT IS YOGA?

DEFINITION OF YOGA

Yoga chitta vritti nirodha (Yoga Sutras 1.2).
When the mind stills yoga occurs.

THE MEANING OF YOGA

Yoga means unity and is derived from the word – yuj, which means to unite in Sanskrit. This unity or connection in the spiritual sense aims to unite individual consciousness with universal consciousness. In practice, this aims to balance and find harmony between body, mind and emotions. A link between body and soul.

THE PURPOSE OF YOGA

He who knows Kundalini knows yoga. The Kundalini, it's said, is coiled like a serpent. He who can induce her to move is liberated (Hatha Yoga Pradipika v.105-111).

The absolute purpose of yoga is to awaken Kundalini Shakti and make her flow. This is a precondition for human evolution. Kundalini Shakti flows in the sushumna nadi along the spine and activates our most important chakras. They are in contact with the brain's untapped resources. When they are used, latent forces are released and we are initiated into the secrets of the universe. We become enlightened and get paranormal abilities – siddhis.

THE GOAL OF YOGA

We can define yoga from a classical perspective; its purpose and meaning, but there is no authority to prescribe what the goal of yoga is – for you. Do you want to reach spiritual goals, get help to rid yourself of back problems or perhaps just be yourself a few minutes a week free from demands and stress?

There is certainly a big difference in the stated goal of yoga if you practice with

Aghori sadhus or among orthodox Hindu swamis. Even greater is the difference between Chinese yoga practitioners and atheists in the Americanized Ashtanga industry. It is and has always been this way. This is the divine essence of yoga. It is as free and amorphous in purpose as in the feeling inside us. Yoga is truly an infinite toolbox. Free to use for what matters most to us. Anandamaya kosha – yoga is unmanifested as our innermost self. When we experience all the power in the universe and on earth – inside and around – we decide for ourselves what the goal of yoga is for us.

THE ORIGIN OF YOGA

The yoga we know today has evolved as part of the Tantric civilization. Some believe the first yogi lived about five-thousand years BCE, others believe that yoga is far older than that.

What we do know is that in the Indus Valley in Harappa and Mohenjodaro (Pakistan), where the pre-Vedic people once lived around 2600 BCE, statues depicting Shiva and Shakti (Parvati) have been found through archaeological excavations.

According to myth, Shiva is the founder of yoga and Parvati is his first disciple. Shiva is seen as a symbol (embodiment) of the highest consciousness. Parvati is considered the mother of the universe. She is the creator and represents knowledge, will, and action. This power, characterized as Kundalini Shakti, is dormant in every human being. Parvati conveyed the secret knowledge of human liberation through tantra. This is where yoga has its roots and from which it cannot be separated, just as consciousness (Shiva) cannot be separated from energy (Shakti).

Yoga probably originated during the beginning of human civilization. Humans began to discover the spiritual potential of man and developed techniques to further develop it. In the past, yoga was kept secret; it was not written down or performed in public. Yoga was passed on orally from guru to student.

Tantric books are the very first to refer to yoga and later also the Vedic scriptures. Rigveda, the oldest Vedic work, was written 3-5000 years BCE, probably by the Indus-Saraswati people. They are a collection of hymns written during a time when the culture in the Indus Valley was flourishing.

According to legend Shiva (pure consciousness) gave yoga to Parvati (Shakti). A fish overheard their conversation and Shiva turned the fish into a human. Not only animals would have yoga but also humans.

VEDIC YOGA / ARCHAIC YOGA

Dating back to 5000 BCE, Vedic yoga is the oldest form of yoga. Sacrifice was seen as a path to the union between inner life, the sensual, and outer life, the material. To practice certain rituals and religions, based on the Vedic hymns (which can be compared to the Old Testament), one had to focus and concentrate for an extended period. To achieve this, yogic techniques were developed. Today this remains the basis of yoga; to use inner focus as a way to increase sensory and human abilities.

Vedic yoga was passed on by rishis (seers), not from guru to student.

PRE-CLASSICAL YOGA

Considered an important work between 2000 BCE to 200 CE, the Upanishads form part of the Vedic scriptures. The Upanishads consist of two hundred Gnostic texts in which yoga is mentioned. Yoga was now taught from guru to student and used to gain insight.

During this time, there were three important yoga paths:

BHAKTI YOGA *– the path of devotion. It refers to devotion to God or the highest consciousness in any of its manifestations. A loving relationship with God is developed through acts such as singing and reciting the name of God. This is seen as the easiest path to moksha.*

JNANA YOGA – *the path of knowledge. In Jnana yoga, insight into and understanding the spiritual aspect is gained by theorizing. Moksha is achieved by understanding that Brahman and atman are the same.*

KARMA YOGA – *the path of selfless action. The practice of selfless action unites practitioners with the highest consciousness. You work and help others without taking credit for it. By being fully present in the work you perform, you become like a tool for the universe.*

The Bhagavad Gita, which can be seen as a summary of the Upanishads, takes place on the battlefield. Krishna tells Arjuna that by following the three yoga paths – Bhakti, Karma and Jnana yoga, he will win the war.

CLASSICAL YOGA

The important work for classical yoga (200CE-400CE) was Patanjali's Yoga Sutras – a verse book and today, one of the six philosophical paths within Hinduism. Yoga now had its philosophy. Patanjali divided yoga into eight steps with a focus on concentration. In this context, asanas meant a stable and comfortable position. The physical body was to be steady and immobile during meditation to avoid distraction.

According to Patanjali, an individual is made up of Prakriti (matter) and Purusha (soul). Here, the goal of yoga is to stop identifying with the corporeal body, and in doing so, the soul will be liberated and allowed to reunite with the Brahman (universe).

POST-CLASSICAL YOGA

All forms of yoga that came into being after Patanjali are categorized as post-classical yoga (500CE-700CE). Here, tantrism has a great influence. Unlike in classical yoga, the body and the mind were now seen as one. Previously, the body had been experienced as an obstacle, and meditation was used as a means to the body and worldly matters. This era focused on returning to the origin of yoga; to rejuvenate the body and learn to master it to awaken Kundalini power. According to tantrism, Kundalini's power exists in every human being, but as a dormant potential. This became the basis of Hatha yoga and the renaissance of tantra. Hatha Yoga Pradipika is an important work in post-classical yoga.

MODERN/CONTEMPORARY YOGA

Swami Vivekananda (1863-1902) was a Hindu theorist and spiritual leader. He was a student of Sri Ramakrishna and founded the Ramakrishna Mission in 1897. There they carried out extensive work in healthcare, provided disaster relief and trained people, among other things. In 1898, Vivekananda attended the World's Fair in the United States where he introduced Hinduism which came to play an important role in the invasion of yoga in the West.

Indra Devi (1899-2001), a German yogi, is another person who played an important role in the development of yoga. Indra is seen as the First Lady of yoga. At the time, yoga was primarily studied and practiced by men. Indra was active in the yoga industry for sixty years; she taught many different nationalities and has been a great inspiration to yogis worldwide. Indra was the first to open a yoga studio in the USA in 1947.

Today's most famous tantric yogi is probably the Dalai Lama.

EVOLUTION OF YOGA THROUGH THE 36 TANTRA TATTWAS

36 TANTRA TATTWAS

Man is an image of the universe. The universe is a macrocosm and man is a microcosm. Everything that is created and that we can see, can also be invisible. It comes down to density and goes from the unmanifested to the manifested.

The thirty-six tantra tattwas describe creation from pure consciousness (Shiva) to matter (Shakti). This is described by thirty-six steps, thirty-six manifestations, of energy that goes from the fine to the rough.

Everything has its beginning in the macrocosm where there is pure consciousness. There was a densification of consciousness/energy. A vibration was heard – spandam, the sound of Aum, and thus Shakti was manifested.

"YOU EXPERIENCE ALL POWER
IN COSMOS AND ON EARTH...

IN YOURSELF AND ALL OVER,
EVERYTHING YOU WANT IS POSSIBLE...

BECAUSE ALL POWER IS YOURS."

5 SHIVA TATTWAS
Macrocosm structure

SHIVA
The timeless; eternal, space

SHAKTI
The manifested; time

ICHA
Will

JNANA
Knowledge

KRIYA
Movement

6 VIDYA TATTWAS

MAYA
Illusion

KALAA
Contraction of KRIYA

VIDYA
Contraction of JNANA

RAGA
Contraction of ICCHA

KALAA
Contraction of Shakti

NIYATI – *contraction CHICCHAKTI (Shiva)*

25 ATMA TATTWAS
Microcosm; man

PURUSHA
Shiva

PRAKRITI
Shakti

BUDDHI – *intellect, insight; SATTVIC GUNA contr. of JNANA*

AHAMKARA – *ego; RAJASIC GUNA contraction of ICCHA*

MANAS – *thoughts; TAMASIC GUNA contraction of KRIYA*

5 st. JNANENDRIYAS
Sound, touch, sight, taste, smell (sense organs, sattvic)

5 st. KARMENDRIYAS
Speech, feeling, walking, emptying (toilet), sneezing (locomotor system, rajasic)

5 st. TANMANTRA
Sound, taste, shape, smell, touch (sensory attributes, tamasic)

5 st. MAHA BHUTAS

PRITHVI
Soil

APAS
Water

AGNI
Fire

VAYU
Air

AKASHA
Space

HATHA YOGA

THE BODY CONTROL OF YOGA

A considerable amount of literature and texts refer to Hatha yoga, most of which were written between 500CE-1400CE of which Hatha Yoga Pradipika by yogi Swatmarama is one of the most famous. References to Hatha yoga are even made in the Upanishads and Puranas, which were written long before the time of Buddhism (about 500 BCE). Traces of Hatha yoga have also been found in pre-Columbian culture in America. Even today there are large stone figures in St. Augustine in South America representing Hatha yoga asanas.

Hatha yoga is associated with Gorakhnath, a leading guru in Hatha yoga (approx. 500 CE-1100 CE). Gorakhnath was a disciple of Matsyendranatha, the first guru in Hatha yoga. Matsya means fish.

Buddha and Mahavir, the founders of the Jain sect, were two important figures in India around 500 BCE. At that time, man's spiritual development had been ongoing for centuries.

Two of the Buddha's teachings became known throughout the world: Vipassana and Anapanasati. For these, the Buddha created a system called the Eightfold Path. This system deals with ethics and correct livelihood, and it has great similarities to Raja yoga's yamas and niyamas. Meditation became a popular method of spiritual development. However, they had no preparatory steps for meditation and eventually began to try the Buddha's system. Meditation was seen as the highest path, but it was acknowledged that some preparations were required before practitioners could sit down to meditate.

Five hundred years after the time of the Buddha, a Buddhist university was established in Nalanda, Bihar, India. It was called the Hinayana system and was an orthodox Buddhist system.

At the same time, another university was established in Vikram Shila, Bihar, India. It became a learning center espousing the Mahayana tradition. They did not agree with the orthodox interpretation of the Buddha's teachings, viewing the Hinayana system as a deviation from the Buddha's teachings. The Mahayana tradition was founded by a group of liberal Buddhists who now began to embrace tantric thinking and philosophy.

After the fall of Buddhism in India (300 CE-500 CE), some great yogis wanted to return to the original doctrine of yoga and tantrism. Matsyendranatha and Goraknatha were two of these. They thought the essence of the doctrine had been forgotten and misunderstood by many. They separated Hatha yoga and Raja yoga from the tantric rituals and developed the most useful, practical exercises in yoga and the tantric system. It also became necessary to reintroduce a proper meditation system. In this way, Hatha yoga was established. Matsyendranatha founded the Natha order.

To cleanse the body and its elements before meditation is the foundation of Hatha yoga.

In Hatha yoga, body and mind are seen as one, and they are equally important.

THE FIVE ELEMENTS OF HATHA YOGA:

ASANAS

In Raja yoga, asanas refer to a comfortable and steady position. In Hatha yoga, asanas are specific postures that help to open up our energy channels and energy centers. Hatha yogis discovered that through good body control, they also gained control over the mind. Therefore, asanas are put at the forefront of Hatha yoga.

PRANAYAMAS

Breathing is used to influence the flow of prana in our nadis (energy channels). Breathwork is a method through which breathing exercises activate, regulate,

*and purify our life energy in the energy body. You get a higher degree of energy
and increase your consciousness.*

MUDRAS

*Mudra can be translated as posture or gesture. Through mudras various energy
points are stimulated, affecting our body and mind. Mudras can be used to
influence your mood and deepen your concentration and consciousness. Through
mudras, you hold on to and redirect prana, which would otherwise disappear
from the body. In this way, mudras also play an important role in awakening
Kundalini Shakti.*

BANDHAS

*Traditionally, bandhas are classified as part of mudras. Bandhas are often
combined with mudras and pranayamas, but they are an important group of
exercises in their own right. Bandha means lock, which describes exercise and its
effect on our energy body. Prana is locked in specific areas of the body and the
flow of prana to the sushumna nadi is controlled, which develops our spiritual
awakening.*

SHATKARMAS

*Shatkarmas are a series of purification processes that are divided into six diffe-
rent groups. The purpose of these is to create harmony between ida and pingala
nadi to achieve mental and physical balance and purity. Purification processes
are also used before breathing exercises to expel toxins from the body.*

HATHA YOGA PRADIPIKA

*Hatha Yoga Pradipika is a classic textbook on Hatha yoga. It was written in the
fifteenth century by Swami Svatmarama who was a disciple of Swami Gorakhnath. Hatha Yoga Pradipika is thus the oldest preserved Hatha yoga text and
one of the three classical texts, next to Gheranda Samhita and Shiva Samhita.*

The book contains a total of three-hundred-and-ninety verses. Of these, about

*forty are dedicated to asanas, about one hundred to pranayamas, one-hund-
red-and-fifty to mudras, bandhas and shatkarmas, and the rest to pratyahara,
dharana, dhyana and samadhi. The book consists of four chapters:*

*1.) Asana: Svatmarama honors his teachers, and explains why he wrote the book
and who he wrote it for. He describes how and where yoga should be practiced.
Svatmarama then describes fifteen asanas and gives recommendations for eating
habits.*

*2.) Pranayama: Svatmarama addresses the connections between breathing,
mind, Kundalini, bandha, nadi and prana. He then describes six karmas and
eight kumbhakas.*

3.) Mudras: The author describes ten different mudras.

*4.) Samadhi: Svatmarama discusses samadhi, laya, nada, two mudras and the
four steps of yoga.*

*Hatha Yoga Pradipika is dedicated to Lord Adinatha, which is another name for
Shiva (a Hindu god of destruction and renewal) and is believed to have revealed
the mysteries of Hatha yoga to his divine consort Parvati.*

HE WHO KNOWS KUNDALINI, KNOWS YOGA

THE KUNDALINI, IT'S SAID,
IS COILED LIKE A SERPENT

HE WHO CAN INDUCE HER TO MOVE
IS LIBERATED

(Hatha Yoga Pradipika v.105-111)

LESSON NO. 1

ASANAS

Basic conditions.

The purpose of Hatha yoga and the performance of different postures is not primarily about how flexible you are or how able you are to get into different positions, but about consciousness. Awareness of the body and breathing. Through this consciousness comes control and through control comes elegance and beauty. The path to achieving the goal of yoga varies and there are many variations on the positions. The most important thing is that the purpose is the same no matter which yoga path you choose.

ATTENTION

Keep your attention on the body. Concentrate on breathing, and become aware of the stretching of muscles and tissues, the movement and the synchronization between breathing and movement. To be able to practice yoga with one's full consciousness in the body, and to turn one's attention inwards is advanced yoga, no matter how simple the exercise is. Hatha yoga practices both the mind and the body.

BREATHING

When performing asanas, make sure that the airways are completely open and clean. The air must be able to pass in and out, without obstacles. Breathe through your nose softly and calmly. When we breathe through the nose, the air is purified and heated before it reaches the throat and lungs. Never hold your breath up at the larynx (glottis and vocal folds). Breathing should be quiet except during certain specific exercises.

IN- AND EXHALE

With the help of inhalation, you can get deeper into certain positions. The inha-

lation creates healthy pressure and stability in the torso e.g. cobra. At the same time, the exhalation helps you to move on and deeper into many other positions, such as in the pliers, for example. In both cases, there are two benefits: breathing with the diaphragm helps you to stretch the tissues in the body and when you pay attention to this, it helps you adjust the position to go deeper.

THE POSITION

Move in and out of position slowly and with full presence. Have an overview of your whole body as you move. Hands, ankles, forearms, elbows, upper arms and shoulders. Feet, ankles, knees, thighs and hips. The pelvis, abdomen, chest, neck and head. In this way, one becomes aware of how the body parts function as a unit. When you learn to move gracefully, it also becomes easier to get into the positions.

PAIN

To avoid injury, you must develop your self-awareness. Before starting a yoga program, it is advisable to try to avoid pain as much as possible. Forcing the body into a position will not only result in injuries but also a state of fear and anxiety. These feelings of fear and anxiety are stored in the nervous system. The body will remember the feeling the next time you do the exercise and it will be harder to get into that position. You should see the pain as a guide who tells you that something is not right. Analyze what feels difficult instead of forcing yourself into the position. With the help of a competent teacher, you can get help finding alternative exercises to get around what feels difficult.

REGULARITY, ENTHUSIASM AND CAUTION

Try to practice at the same time and place every day. This makes it easier to pay attention to differences in how the body feels from day to day. Exercising in the morning is a good basis for improving your health. The stiffness in the morning tells us which parts of the body need the most care and caution. During the day, the body softens and this information is lost, which can lead to becoming injured more easily. Practice with enthusiasm in the morning to counteract stiffness and with caution in the evening to avoid injury. When you start to feel strong and flexible, it is important to be careful as it is easy to go too fast and too deep into a position.

OWN RESPONSIBILITY

In Hatha yoga, there are many asanas where one stands in positions that do not feel natural to the body. These positions reveal the condition of the body and you must decide for yourself if you want to continue entering a position. A good criterion to follow is that it should feel good in the body not just a few hours after the program but also the day after.

It is important to respect the contraindications described for each position and program.

BUILD UP YOUR PATIENCE

Take your time. Cultivate patience and make progress gradually. Be present in the experience and enjoy the moment no matter what and let go of all expectations of results.

THINGS TO THINK ABOUT BEFORE THE LESSON

Pay extra attention to whether someone suffers from high blood pressure, for example, or any other disease that should be taken into account.

Stay for a long time in the end position and the shavasana. At least about 2-3 min.

Keep track of the pace, do not increase the pace if it does not feel natural.

Do not encourage achievement in beginner classes.

Instruct breathing before execution/entry position.

No extreme "hold your breath" in the breathing exercises. Guide by saying: "Breath in, wait for exhalation and exhale".

Give clear instructions when you start with a new exercise: "Sit up, we will now practice" ... " Lie down, we will..."

Always end the asanas with a few moments lying in the shavasana for rest/contemplation.

Have some water with you (you quickly get a dry throat when you lead a lesson) and a watch on hand to make it easier to keep track of time. 2-5 min is enough time in each asana in the beginning.

Be careful to show any alternative asanas before starting the class, for example, a pillow and vajrasana.

ADVICE FOR PERFORMING THE ASANAS

BREATH
It is important to breathe through the nose (unless otherwise stated) and coordinate the breathing with the movement.

CONSCIOUSNESS
The purpose of asanas is to influence and create harmony in all aspects of man. Physically, mentally, emotionally, pranic and spiritually. By performing asanas consciously, one can affect all these parts. One should be aware of body sensations, movement, positioning and coordination with the breathing, the flow of prana, focus on the chakra and acknowledge thoughts and feelings that come up.

RELAXATION
You can lie down in the shavasana at any time for rest/contemplation and be aware of how it feels in the body.

SERIES

*You always start with shatkarma (purification processes) e.g. nasal rinsing –
then perform asanas, pranayamas, pratyahara and dharana (concentration/
quiet mind) which leads to dhyana (meditation). You can also do both breathing exercises and meditation before the asanas, but it fulfills a function at the
beginning of your yoga practice that you go from the outside to the inside. See
the text about our five bodies before you intuitively know what, when and how
to practice.*

OPPOSITION

*It is important to have a structure in the program to balance the body and
nervous system. A forward bending position should always be followed by a
backward bending position and vice versa. However, this does not apply to yoga
rehabilitation.*

TIME

*Asanas can be practiced at any time of the day, provided you have not eaten
a few hours before. However, it is recommended to practice two hours before
sunrise or just before sunset. The time before sunrise is called Brahma muhurta.
The atmosphere is then clean and still, the stomach and intestines inactive and
the mind still.*

PLACE

*One should find a private place where it is tidy, clean, quiet and peaceful. No
furniture or objects should be in the way. You can also practice outdoors in a
comfortable and beautiful place. However, not in a cold or windy spot or where
the air is unclean.*

CARPET

*Use a base of natural material. It has the most beneficial effect on our pranic
currents.*

CLOTHES

Wear loose and comfortable clothes and take off your jewelry.

SHOWER

Try to take a cold shower before yoga to wake up the body.

TOILET

It is recommended that you visit the bathroom before beginning your practice.

DIET

There are no strict rules for what food to eat. However, a natural diet in moderate amounts is recommended so that not all energy is used to digest the food. A vegetarian diet is not essential but is recommended. The stomach should be half filled with food, a quarter with water and a quarter should be left empty.

EXECUTION AND GUIDANCE

Asanas are performed gently in three steps:

Awareness of the body, the movement and thoughts that emerge. This creates calm, balance and focus, which in turn leads to a state of harmony in the body.

Awareness of breathing. Synchronize the movement with the breathing. The movement becomes calmer and brain waves slower. You become relaxed and gain an increased awareness.

Awareness of the flow of prana. You may experience this as a tingling in the body. You can develop the feeling through regular practice. You achieve mental calmness and become focused and emotionally receptive.

Asanas are also divided into three parts:

Starting position.

Implementation.

End position.

LEADING THE CLASS

A good way to start the exercises is to say: "We start with that" ... and then ... "with the next exhalation we can finish and come back on e.g. back".

Encourage students to stretch, lengthen the spine on inhalation, and maintain the stretch on exhalation. Pull down the shoulders so that there is as long a distance as possible between the ears and shoulders. To breathe from the stomach. Experience the body from the inside, experience the body before and after each position. Pay attention to consciousness.

The pedagogy we use is called **VAK:**

Visual. Auditory. Kinesthetic.

See. Hear. Do.

Show. Explain + show. To lead-in.

Show first (can everyone see?).

Then explain (can everyone hear?).

Lead in (starting position: "We sit in the starting position, breathe in ...")

Perform (possibly at everyone's own pace).

Exit (at the same time: "We end with the next exhalation ...")

Starting position (explore bodily sensations: "How does it feel in the body ...")

IMPORTANT

In the event of any injury or illness, a physician should be consulted before performing the asanas. Your joints, hard parts or ligaments must never hurt whilst carrying out the asanas.

Inverted asanas should be avoided if feeling gassy (toxins may sink into the brain), during late pregnancy or menstruation (the cycle may be disrupted).

You should never sunbathe or swim immediately after yoga due to the risk of overheating.

YOGA CLASS FOR BEGINNERS

The lesson is estimated to take about 45-60 minutes in addition to the deep relaxation and meditation at the end. Have a clock in front of you so you can keep track of time. If there is no breathing exercise at the beginning of the beginner's session, we can spend a little longer in long shavasana instead. The participants must be allowed to "land" and unwind on their backs before starting with the positions. Do not rush through any exercise. If you notice that you are short on time, delete a sequence instead. Have a glass of water in front of you so you do not get a dry throat. Speak slowly, clearly and loudly. Get to know the students, be observant of all movements and check that everyone is present in what they are doing. Encourage students to close their eyes and focus on the exercise and what is happening in the body. Encourage awareness and presence. A good way to start the exercises is to say – we start with...and end with – with the next exhalation, we can end and come back on e.g. back. You will learn yoga nidra in module 3.

LONG SHAVASANA - DEAD MAN´S POSTURE/RELAXATION.
PRANAYAMA – YOGIC BREATHING.
SUPTA PAWANMUKTASANA – LEG LOCK.

MARJARIASANA – THE CAT.

NAUKA SANCHALANA – ROWING THE BOAT.

JANU SIRSHASANA – PREPARATORY BACK STRETCH.

KANDHARASANA – SHOULDER POSE.

SHAVASANA – DEAD MAN´S POSTURE.

SHAVA UDARAKARSHANASANA – THE UNIVERSAL POSITION.

SHAVASANA – DEAD MAN´S POSTURE.

SARPASANA – THE SNAKE.

SHASHANKASANA – THE HARE.

SHAVASANA – DEAD MAN´S POSTURE.

YOGA NIDRA – DEEP RELAXATION.

END WITH - HARI OM TAT SAT, 3 TIME.

THEN - OM SRI DURGAYAI NAMAH, 1 TIME.

LONG SHAVASANA

We begin all lessons with a long relaxation in shavasana. Let the participants lie on their backs, facing you so they can hear better.

You can have the text in front of you on the floor until you know it by heart.

YOU START WITH COMMON SHAVASANA

Lie down comfortably on your back ...

Let your legs and arms relax away from your body. Breathe through your nose and turn your palms upwards, then bring your chin down towards your chest and close your eyes ...

THEN YOU CONTINUE WITH THE LONG SHAVASANA

Feel the different parts of your body in contact with the floor ...

Take your consciousness to your right leg ... feel the contact between your right calf and the floor ... feel the contact between your right heel and the floor ... relax the whole right leg ...

Take your consciousness to your left leg ... feel the contact between your left calf and the floor ... feel the contact between your left heel and the floor ... relax the entire left leg ...

Now take your consciousness to the posterior ... feel the contact between the buttocks and the floor ... relax the buttocks ... relax both legs and let them sink deep into the floor ...

Move your attention to your right arm ... feel the contact between your right arm and the floor ... the contact between your right hand and the floor ... relax the whole right arm.

Move your attention to your left arm ... feel the contact between your left arm and the floor ... the contact between your left hand and the floor ... relax the whole left arm ...

Be aware of the contact between your shoulder blades and the floor ... relax your whole back ... let your shoulders sink into the floor ... feel the contact between the back of your head and the floor ... relax your neck, forehead, eyes, cheeks, lips, tongue, lower jaw, face ... your whole body is completely relaxed and feels heavy ...

The whole right leg is heavy and sinks deep into the floor ... the left leg also sinks into the floor ... your shoulders, head, left and right arm also sink deeper into the floor ...

Each time you breathe, your body sinks deeper into the floor ... with each exhalation, your body becomes heavier and heavier ...

TERMINATION

Hari Om Tat Sat 3 times.

...we can open our eyes and start moving our bodies ...

INSTRUCTIONS FOR ASANAS LESSON NO 1.

LONG SHAVASANA – DEAD MAN'S POSTURE/RELAXATION. *5-10 min.*

PRANAYAMA– YOGIC BREATHING.

Execution: Place one hand on the stomach and one hand on the chest to begin with. Inhale, fill your stomach like a balloon, then fill your chest – at the front, under your arms and into the back, hold your breath at the collarbones (use the chin to hold your breath), then release your breath – first from your chest and then your stomach. Empty your lungs (bahir kumbhaka) and then start again. 5-10 min.

SUPTA PAWANMUKTASANA – LEG LOCK.

Execution: Lie on your back with your legs touching and your arms alongside your body. Inhale and lift the right leg, exhale, bend the leg, clasp your hands around the knee and pull the leg towards the upper body. On one exhale, lift your head and bring your chin up towards your knee. Press the left leg into the mat. Stay and breathe. Exhale and bring your head down, inhale, stretch out your right leg, exhale and bring your leg down. Do the same with the left leg. 2-3 min.

MARJARIASANA – THE CAT.

Execution: Kneel on all fours. Place your hands directly underneath your shoulders and your knees directly underneath your hips. Keep your back and neck straight and look down at the floor. Exhale, arch your back. Inhale, return to the starting position.. 2-3 min.

NAUKA SANCHALANA – ROWING THE BOAT.

Execution: Sit with straight legs and grab your thumbs. Inhale - clench your fists as if they were holding oars, exhale and extend your hands towards your feet. Keep your knees soft in the extended position so that your lumbar spine is protected. 2-3 min.

JANU SIRSHASANA – PREPARATORY BACK STRETCH.

Execution: Sit with both legs straight out in front of you, preferably on the edge of a folded blanket so that your pelvis tilts slightly forward. Bend the right leg and place the sole of the right foot high up against the left inner thigh. Inhale, straighten your back and fold forward keeping your back straight. Push your chest forward. Place a belt around your left foot to help pull yourself forward. Then bend forward and try to get your head towards your foot. Grasp the foot if it is available to you, otherwise, use the belt. Inhale and roll up. Repeat on the other side. 2-3 min.

KANDHARASANA – SHOULDER POSTURE.

Execution: Lie on your back and bend your knees. Keep your feet wide apart and your soles flat on the floor. Grab your ankles. Inhale and push your buttocks up as high as you can toward the ceiling. Hold your breath for as long as you can. When you get tired, go down and rest/breathe and then see if you can push up a little higher next time on an inhalation. 2-3 min.

SHAVASANA – DEAD MAN'S POSTURE.

Execution: Move the legs slightly apart, let your feet fall to the sides and lie with the arms slightly away from the body. Turn your palms upwards. Stretch your spine, tip your chin down and breathe deeply with your stomach. Concentrate on your breathing and feel the whole body from the inside out to completely relax. 2-3 min.

SHAVA UDARAKARSHANASANA – THE UNIVERSAL POSITION.

Execution: Lie on your back, lift your right leg and bend at the knee. Place the left hand on the right knee, exhale and pull the knee over to the left side. Extend your right arm out at a 90-degree angle to your body and turn your head to look at your right hand. Try to push the right shoulder blade into the mat. Stay here and breathe in and out. Inhale and roll back onto your back. Repeat on the left side. 2-3 min. on each side.

SARPASANA – THE SNAKE.

Execution: Lie on your stomach and keep your chin on the mat. Clasp your hands behind your back. Inhale, lift your upper back and stretch your arms back towards your feet. Hold and breathe. Exhale and slowly lower back down to the mat. 2-3 min.

SHASHANKASANA – THE HARE.

Execution: This pose is recommended after backbends. Lie on your stomach, put your hands under your shoulders and push yourself back so you sit on your heels, lean forward with your forehead touching the floor and stretch your arms out in front. Stay here and breathe in and out. Become aware of your breathing. 2-3 min.

AJNA CHAKRA (READ ABOUT THE CHAKRA IN MODULE 4)

To practice regularly for a month.

Chakra and kshetram localization /activation and purification through Shambhavi mudra with Om chanting (open eyes – fast Om, then close your eyes and inhale slowly – O … in through bhrumadhya (eyebrow center) … out with M …) Experience the pulsation from the chakra and visualize the color. You can also visualize the yantra.

Anuloma viloma pranayama alt. prana shuddhi. Inhale through the left nostril and exhale through the right nostril and count to 1. Inhale through the right nostril and out through the left and count to 1. Inhale through the left nostril and count to 2, exhale through the right and count to 2. Etc. On 5, 10 and 15 etc. you inhale through both and out through both nostrils. If you lose the count, you start again from 1.

Trataka. Light a candle and sit in a meditation position with a straight back. Squint at the light, do not fully close your eyes. Look at the embers in the flame for 30 seconds, then close your eyes and look at the after-image of the flame behind your closed eyes …

KNOWLEDGE TEST MODULE 1

ANSWER AS FULLY AS YOU CAN, THEN CHECK IF YOU ANSWERED CORRECTLY. PRACTICE UNTIL YOU KNOW THE ANSWERS BY HEART.

1. WHAT IS YOGA'S DEFINITION IN SANSKRIT AND ENGLISH?

2. DESCRIBE THE ORIGIN OF YOGA.

3. WHAT IS CLASSICAL YOGA?

4. WHAT DO THE 36 TANTRIC TATTWAS SYMBOLIZE?

5. DESCRIBE HATHA YOGA AND ITS ORIGINS.

6. WHAT ARE THE FIVE PARTS WHICH HATHA YOGA IS DIVIDED INTO?

7. WHAT SHOULD BE CONSIDERED WHEN PERFORMING ASANAS?

8. WHAT IS VAK?

9. DESCRIBE AJNA CHAKRA, ITS ELEMENT, YANTRA, COLOR, NUMBER OF PETALS AND ATTRIBUTES.

10. DESCRIBE SOME POWERFUL EXERCISES TO ACTIVATE, CLEAN AND BALANCE AJNA CHAKRA.

MODULE 2

WE STUDY HATHA YOGA FROM A PRACTICAL PERSPECTIVE AND DEEPEN OUR THEORETICAL KNOWLEDGE

We study purification processes (shatkarma), the most important postures (asana), breathing exercises (pranayama), postures (mudras), locks (bandhas) and get an orientation in the pranic (energy) body. We study the Mooladhara chakra and practice our exercises to cleanse, balance and activate the chakra. We continue to practice in the role of yoga teacher with lesson no. 2 of 8.

Knowledge test: Answer the questions that relate to module 2. Practice lesson no. 2 with at least 1 participant and humbly accept feedback from them. Ask questions afterward – how was the pace, did you keep to time, did you speak loudly enough, and how well did you understand the exercises?

ADVANCED HATHA YOGA

OUR FIVE SHEATHS

Our physical body, the three bodies of the astral body and our innermost interior.

Hatha yoga teaches that we consist of five sheaths or bodies:

ANNAMAYA KOSHA

Physical body.

PRANAMAYA KOSHA

Energy body.

MANAMAYA KOSHA

Mental body.

VIGYANAMAYA KOSHA

Wisdom body

ANANDAMAYA KOSHA

Bliss body (pure consciousness of true self).

The energy body, the mental body and the wisdom body form the astral body.

NADIS – IDA AND PINGALA AND SUSHUMNA NADI

Pranamaya kosha – our energy body – consists of about seventy-two thousand nadis (subtle channels through which prana flows). It is the energy body that gives us life. The three most important nadis are ida, pingala and sushumna nadi of which sushumna nadi is the most important.

Ida nadi flows from the left side of the spine and controls mental energy. It is associated with the parasympathetic nervous system. Pingala nadi flows along the right side of the spine and controls our physical body. It is associated with the sympathetic nervous system. Sushumna nadi, the most important of the three, flows along the entire spine and channels the spiritual energy.

Ida and pingala nadi flow from the root chakra and cross the sushumna nadi at four places in the body to finally unite at the eyebrow center. Ida nadi then goes out through the left nostril and pingala nadi through the right.

We can regulate the body's energies through asanas, and when ida and pingala nadi flow simultaneously, sushumna nadi opens. Kundalini Shakti can begin to travel upwards and activate our chakra system, thereby illuminating the parts of our brain that are dormant. Usually, we use about twenty percent of our brain capacity. On our path to activating a larger part of the brain special siddhis, paranormal abilities, arise. You become a Siddha. However, these abilities are not the ultimate goal.

HA + THA

Ha – pingala nadi – the sun stands for the sympathetic nervous system, and tha – ida nadi – the moon stands for the parasympathetic nervous system.

OUR SUBTLE ENERGY BODY WITH FIVE PRANA VAYUS

Our five bodies interact with each other and create a whole. The breathing exercises mainly affect our energy body – pranamaya kosha, which is made up of five different types of sub-pranas. These five prana vayus (wind) are prana, apana, samana, udana and vyana. It is also the link that binds the bodies together and affects us in all directions. If we calm the body with breathing, we also calm the mind and vice versa, which you probably have experienced during your yoga practice.

PRANA

In this context, prana does not refer to the cosmic prana, but to the flow of energy that controls the area of the thorax between the larynx and the diaphragm. This area is linked to the heart and respiratory system along with the muscles and nerves that activate them. It is this power that makes us draw inward breath.

APANA

Apana controls the abdomen and the area under the navel, and it provides energy to the intestines, kidneys, rectum and genitals. It affects the expulsion of waste products in the body and is the force that makes us exhale.

SAMANA

Samana is located between the heart and the navel. It activates and controls the digestive system. Samana is responsible for the transformation; physically, the transformation refers to the very distribution of nutrients in the body, and evolutionarily, it refers to Kundalini power and the development of our consciousness.

UDANA

Udana controls the area of the neck and head. It activates all our sensory receptors such as eyes, tongue, nose and ears. Udana activates and creates a balance in muscles, ligaments, nerves and joints in our arms and legs. It is responsible for our posture, our sensory attention and our ability to interact with the outside world.

VYANA

Vyana permeates the whole body. It regulates and controls all our movements and coordinates all sub-pranas in the body.

In addition to the most important sub-pranas, there are also five smaller pranas called upa-pranas. These five are naga, koorma, krikara, devadatta and dhananjaya. Naga is responsible for belching and hiccups, koorma opens our eyes and makes us blink, krikara creates hunger, thirst, sneezing and coughing, devadatta generates sleep and yawning, and dhananjaya activates when we die and our body begins to break down.

PRANA AND LIFESTYLE

Our lifestyle has a big impact on our energy body and its prana. Physical activity such as exercise, work, sleep, food, and sexual relationships affect the distribution and flow of prana in our body. Emotions, thoughts, and fantasies affect our bodies even more. An unbalanced lifestyle, poor diet, and stress break down and block the flow of prana. It results in feeling drained of energy. When energy becomes low in one of our sub-pranas, the very area of the body that the prana controls is affected and may result in illness. Breathing exercises can prevent this by balancing or increasing the energy in our energy body.

ASANA

There is a definition of asanas – Stirham Sukham Asana – in Patanjali's Yoga Sutras which means steady or comfortable position. They wanted to develop their ability to sit still for a long time because it was a prerequisite for meditation.

In Hatha yoga, however, it was discovered that certain postures, asanas, opened up energy channels and mental centers in the body. You got better body control and could thus also develop control over the mind, thoughts, and energies. Yoga asanas became a tool for achieving higher consciousness and provided the stable foundation required to explore the body, mind and breathing.

Originally, there were eight-million-four-hundred-thousand different asanas. These represent as many lives as an unenlightened person must be reborn into before he becomes enlightened. Rishis and yogis scaled down the number to the few hundred known today. Of these, the eighty-four most important asanas were then highlighted. Thirty-five asanas have a direct impact on our chakras. The others purify and regulate our nadis. Asanas create a balance between body and mind, and a flow in the sushumna.

Rishis studied the animals and noticed how they lived in harmony with their body and surroundings. By mimicking the animals' movements and postures, hormone secretion in the body was affected. During deep meditation, they were able to observe how different postures affected both the body and the mind.

Prana, the vital energy (life energy), permeates our entire body. Poor flow of prana in the body results in stiffness and an accumulation of toxins. When prana flows freely, these toxins are removed and the body becomes soft and supple. Even the most difficult postures are easy to perform. When the amount of prana increases in the body, pranic intuition is achieved. An intuitive sense of how to perform asanas, mudras and pranayamas follows.

Hatha yoga not only increases overall health but also activates our energy centers by balancing the nervous system.

Asanas in Hatha yoga release tensions that arise as knots in our muscles. By releasing these tensions from the body, we also release tensions from the mind. It makes us feel better in general and releases underlying and hidden energy that lies latent.

Thus asanas are more than just exercise. They are techniques that place the body in different positions to promote awareness, relaxation, concentration and meditation. Part of this process is to develop a good physique through stretching, stimulation of prana, and massage of the glands and internal organs.

Asanas are divided into three groups: beginners, intermediate and advanced. It is not necessary to complete all the exercises in each group. Daily practice of a tailor-made program will have the greatest effect.

Asanas for beginners should be performed by those who have never practiced yoga before. These have a greater effect on the body in beginners than in advanced exercises. These exercises prepare the body and mind for more advanced exercises as well as meditation and are very useful for improving physical health.

The intermediate asanas are for those who can complete the exercises for beginners without difficulty. These require greater concentration, steadiness and coordination in connection with movement and breathing.

Advanced asanas are for those who have well-developed body control, muscles and nervous system. You should be able to master the intermediate exercises without problem. It is important not to rush and start these exercises too early.

DYNAMIC AND STATIC ASANAS

Dynamic asanas increase flexibility and circulation in the body. They soften muscles, release knots and energy blockages, and remove stagnant blood. These asanas are most important for the beginner. To be able to work with the chakra system, for example, blockages must first be released, otherwise, the energy may flow the wrong way in the energy body. Dynamic asanas and vinyasa process our physical body; they take us deeper and prepare us for the more static asanas. Hatha yoga often starts with a lot of movement and then gradually lets the vibrations subside into stillness and silence. This also has a lot to do with us moving from the rough to the fine – from the body to the mind – and the knowledge of how yoga affects our doshas through Ayurveda.

VINYASA

Dynamic asanas are often synchronized with breathing. When we do that, it's called vinyasa. A flow where movements and breathing interact.

Vinyasa aims to increase the internal cleansing and detoxification of the body. Breathing synchronized with movement warms the blood. Thick blood is often unhealthy and causes diseases. The heat from vinyasa cleanses the blood and makes it thinner so it can circulate better in the body, and around our joints, and reduce any pain.

Where there is poor circulation in the body, pain usually occurs. The heated blood also passes through all the internal organs, and transports impurities and diseases away that are removed from the body with our increased amount of sweat during the yoga session.

Sweat is an important by-product of vinyasa. It is only through our sweat that diseases can leave the body and be purified, in the same way, that gold is melted to get rid of its impurities. Yoga boils the blood and transports impurities and toxins to the surface, which are then removed with the help of sweat. If you practice vinyasa often, the body becomes healthy and strong, and clean and shiny like gold.

With the body cleansed, it is possible to cleanse the nervous system and sense organs.

STATIC ASANAS

Static and, above all, inverted asanas have the deepest effect on our energy body and our chakra system. These require greater flexibility and are suited for more experienced practitioners. Remaining in the position for a few minutes gives a more powerful effect on the glands, prana, chakras and internal organs. The mind becomes calm and prepares the individual for meditation. Some static asanas are very useful for reaching pratyahara.

TRISTHANA

Tristhana means three areas to pay attention to: postures (position, stretching and relaxation), breath and gazing point. They are always performed in conjunction with each other.

Asanas cleanse, strengthen and soften the body. When we breathe with rechaka and puraka, a steady and even inhalation and exhalation at the same pace, we cleanse the nervous system. Drishti is the place you look at during yoga practice. There are nine different ones: the tip of the nose, eyebrow center, navel, thumbs, hands, feet, right and left side, up to the sky. Drishi purifies, captures and stabilizes the mind.

ADVICE FOR THE PRACTICE OF ASANAS:

BREATH

According to Hatha yoga, two components are needed to cleanse the body internally: the elements air and fire. Fire, our life force, is located at the solar plexus in the body and is generated by the Manipura chakra. Air is required for fire to burn, hence the importance of proper breathing in yoga. Long, even breaths increase the internal fire, agnin, in the body, which in turn heats up the blood for physical purification and burns up impurities in the nervous system. As the internal fire increases in strength, so does our digestive system, health and longevity. Uneven breathing creates an imbalance in both our physical body and its signaling system, weakening our immune system. We risk becoming ill in the long run – according to Hatha yoga, we tolerate both stress and toxins less.

Another important component to increase the inner fire is to use moola and uddiyana bandha: root and stomach locks. They increase the effect of breathing, keep it inside the body longer, encapsulate the energy, and provide light, strength and health to the body. According to Hatha yoga, there are six toxins in the body that surround our spiritual heart. The light in our heart is obscured by these six poisons: kama, krodha, moha, lobha, matsarya, and mada. They are desire, anger, delusion, greed, envy and sloth. When we have practiced Hatha yoga for an extended period with power, determination and the right breathing, the increasing heat in the body will burn up these six toxins and the light in our interior will shine through.

It is important to breathe through the nose (unless otherwise stated) and coordinate breathing with movement. But never force yourself to breathe through your nose. If you need to breathe through your mouth, do it. Your fine energy channels can be damaged otherwise and the energy will flow the wrong way in the energy body. If you are panting, wait until you can breathe through your nose again without greater difficulty.

CONSCIOUSNESS

The purpose of asanas is to influence and create harmony in all aspects of man: physical, mental, emotional, pranic and spiritual. By performing asanas consciously, all these parts are affected. One should be aware of body sensations, movement, and posture on its own and in coordination with breathing, the flow of prana, focus on chakra and witness thoughts and feelings that come up.

RELAXATION

You can lie down in shavasana at any time for rest or contemplation. Notice how it feels in the body.

SERIES

You always begin with shatkarmas (purification processes) such as nasal rinsing (jala neti), then you perform asanas, pranayamas, pratyahara and dharana (concentration/quiet the mind) which lead to dhyana (meditation). You can also add both breathing exercises and meditation before asanas. It fulfills a function – especially at the beginning of your yoga practice, that you go from the outside in (see the text about our five bodies) before you intuitively know what, when and how to do.

OPPOSITION

It is important to have a structure in the program to balance the body and nervous system. A forward bending position should always be followed by a backward bending position and vice versa. However, this does not apply to yoga rehabilitation.

TIME

Asanas can be practiced at any time of the day, provided you have not eaten a few hours prior. With that said, it is recommended to practice just before sunrise and sunset. The time of day just before sunrise is called Brahma muhurta (the divine time – God's time). The atmosphere is clean and still then, the stomach and intestines inactive and the mind still. The most favorable time is before sun-

rise and before sunset, but do not be too ambitious from the outset. It is better to have a yoga session during the day than no session at all.

PLACE

One should find a secluded place where it is tidy, clean, quiet and peaceful. No furniture or objects should be in the way. You can also practice outdoors in a comfortable and beautiful place. However, not in the cold and wind, where the air is unclean or in the scorching sun.

CARPET

Use a base of natural materials. It has the most beneficial effect on our pranic currents.

CLOTHES

Wear loose and comfortable clothes, remove jewelry, and be barefoot so you do not slip.

SHOWER

Try to take a cold shower before the session to wake the body up. After the session, wait to shower so you do not cool down your body too quickly and lose the healing effect of yoga unnecessarily.

LOO

Empty the stomach.

DIET

There are no strict rules regulating what food to eat. However, a natural diet in moderate amounts is recommended so that not all energy is used to digest food. A vegetarian diet is not essential but it is recommended. The stomach should be filled half with food, a quarter with water and a quarter should be left empty. However, do not drink water during the practice as it draws blood and energy to the stomach and cools down your energy body. As you know, we want to get the energy out of the body during yoga. Also, wait two to three hours to practice yoga after you have eaten so it does not feel uncomfortable during the session.

PERFORMANCE

Asanas are performed softly and gently in three steps:

Awareness of the body, movement and thoughts that arise. This creates calm, balance and focus, which in turn leads to a state of harmony in the body.

Awareness of breathing. Synchronize movement with breathing. The movement becomes calmer and brain waves slower. You become relaxed and gain an increased awareness.

Awareness of the flow of prana. It can be experienced as tingles in the body. The feeling is developed through regular practice. You become mentally calm, focused, and emotionally receptive.

Asanas are also divided into three parts:

Starting poses.
Implementation.
Final poses.

IMPORTANT

In the event of any injury or illness, a physician should be consulted before performing asanas.

Asanas must never hurt joints, hard parts or ligaments during practice.

Inverted asanas should be avoided during gas formation (toxins can reach the brain), late pregnancy, and menstruation (the cycle can be disrupted). Never sunbathe immediately following yoga practice to avoid overheating.

PRANAYAMA

*Pranayama means breathing technique or breathing control and originates
from the words prana – (life force or life energy), yama (discipline or control),
and ayama (extension, restraint or expansion). Pranayamas are divided into
puraka (inhalation), kumbhaka (retention of breath), and rechaka (exhalation).
Kumbhaka, in turn, is divided into bahir (the retention of breath immediately
following exhalation) and antar (holding your breath inside after inhaling).
In yogic writings, kevala kumbhaka is also mentioned. It is an advanced yogic
condition where breathing via the lungs stops spontaneously and energy (prana)
seeps through the pores in the body's cells.*

HEALTH AND BREATHING

*Breathing is the most important function we have in the body. It affects the
activity of every single cell, including the brain and its functions. A person bre-
athes about fifteen breaths per minute and about twenty-thousand-six hundred
breaths per day. Most of us breathe incompletely, using only a small part of our
lungs' capacity. The breathing then becomes shallow and the body becomes poor
in oxygen and prana, which are necessary to maintain good health.*

*Rhythmic, deep and slow breathing encourages and is encouraged by a calm
and satisfied state of mind. Irregular and uneven breathing disrupts the rhythm
of the brain which leads to physical, emotional, and mental blockages. This, in
turn, cause internal conflicts, an unbalanced personality, a disordered lifestyle,
and illness. Through breathing exercises, you build up a regular breathing
pattern and break this vicious circle. We learn to regain control of our breathing
and rebuild the natural, relaxed rhythm of our body and mind.*

*Despite being an unconscious process, you can turn breathing into a conscious
process at any time. This creates a link between the unconscious and conscious
parts of our mind. The energy that is absorbed by neurotic and unconscious
mental patterns can be released with the help of breathing exercises. The energy
can then be used on something creative and joyful.*

BREATHING AND LIFE

Ancient yogis and rishis studied nature in detail. They noted that animals with slow breathing had a long lifespan and animals with fast breathing only lived for a few years. Through this observation, they realized how important slow breathing is for longevity. Physically, breathing is directly linked to the heart. Slow breathing keeps the heart strong which leads to a longer life. Deep breathing also increases the absorption of energy in our energy body which increases mobility, vitality and well-being.

BREATHING EXERCISES AND THE SPIRITUAL SEARCH

Breathing exercises build a healthy body by releasing blockages in the energy body, and this increases the absorption and retention of prana in the body. A calm and quiet mind is a prerequisite for spiritual exercises. In many breathing exercises, kumbhaka (retention of breath) is used to control the flow of prana, calm the mind, and control the thought process. When the mind is calmed down and prana can flow freely through our nadis and chakras, the development of our consciousness is enabled. This, in turn, can lead us to higher dimensions of spiritual experiences.

COMMON ADVICE

Contraindications. Breathing exercises should not be practiced during illness. However, lighter exercises such as conscious breathing or abdominal breathing in shavasana are still acceptable.

TIME

The best time for breathing exercises is in the morning before the sun rises. The body is calm and the mind is still, as it has not yet had time to absorb many impressions from its surroundings. If this is not possible, the second-best time is in the evening when the sun goes down. Soothing breathing exercises are good to do before falling asleep. Try to do the breathing exercises at the same time and in the same place every day. Regular practice builds strength and willpower.

HYGIENE

Take a bath or shower before practicing pranayamas. At least, wash hands, face and feet. Wait at least half an hour to bathe after completing breathing exercises. This is to allow the body temperature to normalize.

FOOD

Eat your breakfast after completing the practice or wait three to four hours after eating to practice. With food in the stomach, pressure is formed on the diaphragm and lungs, which makes it difficult to breathe deeply and completely. It hinders the use of the full capacity of the lungs.

When you start practicing breathing exercises, you may experience constipation and a decrease in urine. If this occurs, reduce salt and spices, and drink plenty of water. Should you instead experience an anxious stomach and an increase in urine, take a break from practice for a few days.

PLACE

Practice in a place where you can find peace, and where it is clean. The place should be well-ventilated, but not so that you are sitting in a draft. Avoid direct sunlight as it may cause overheating.

BREATH

Always breathe through your nose unless otherwise instructed. The air must be able to flow freely through both nostrils.

SEQUENCE

Breathing exercises are done after shatkarmas and often after asanas, and before meditation, but can also be practiced before asanas. Nadi shodana should be included in each breathing exercise. Lie down in shavasana for a few minutes after completing the exercises.

SITTING POSITION

A comfortable sitting position is necessary to be able to keep the body and breathing stable during the exercises. The body should be as relaxed as possible with a straight spine and neck. The seat pad should be made of natural material. If you cannot sit comfortably in a meditation position for a long time, you can sit against a wall with outstretched legs or on a chair with a straight backrest.

Avoid exertion. It is important to remember not to exert too much effort when doing breathing exercises. Do not be in a hurry to advance. Do not move on to the next step until you feel fully comfortable with an exercise. Keeping your breath inside/out is only achieved as long as it feels comfortable.

SIDE EFFECTS

Various physical and mental symptoms can occur in normally healthy people. Physical symptoms occur as a result of the detoxification of toxins. Feelings such as tingling, heat and cold, lightness and heaviness may occur. These are usually temporary. Energy levels may increase or fluctuate, and interests may change. If these changes create problems, you should seek the guidance of a competent guru. Excessive pranayamas late at night can lead to sleeping problems as well as an extreme excess of energy the next day – what many wrongly describe as a Kundalini awakening or hypersensitivity. Pranayamas are powerful tools and should be treated with respect. Slightly simplified, you can say that through breathing exercises agni (fire) is increased in us, and Manipura chakra at the navel increases its activity. This causes vayu (air) attached to the chakra above, Anahata, to be netted and expanded. As the air expands, so does the space within us (akasha) and a deeper spiritual experience is reached. However, increasing the amount of vayu can lead to anxiety and worry, so you must end each session by reducing the excess of vata you have built up. Excessive practice can, in the worst case, lead to psychosis and delusions.

MUDRA/GESTURE

Mudra can be translated as posture or gesture. Through mudras, various energy points that affect both body and mind are stimulated. Your mood is influenced and your consciousness and ability to concentrate are increased. With the help of mudras, you can hold and control prana that would otherwise disappear from the body. Hence, mudras also play an important role in awakening Kundalini energy. Mudras can be done as a single exercise or in combination with asanas, pranayamas, bandhas and different visualization techniques.

In Hatha Yoga Pradipika, mudras are discussed as "yoganaga" : a separate bran-ch of yoga that requires a subtle presence. You often learn these techniques after you have become accustomed to and knowledgeable in asanas, pranayamas, bandhas, and when you have eliminated blockages from the body. Mudras are among the more advanced techniques that awaken our prana, chakranas and Kundalini Shakti, which in turn can open up various siddhis (paranormal or mental forces) in the more advanced practitioners.

Mudras create a direct link between annamaya kosha (our physical body), manomaya kosha (our mental body) and pranamaya kosha (our energy body). This increases the feeling and awareness of the flow of prana in the body. A pranic balance is created in our koshas and the subtle energy is directed to the higher chakras, which promotes an increased degree of consciousness.

Our nadis and chakras radiate energy which normally disappears from the body into our surroundings. By creating barriers within the body with the help of mudras, the energy is instead directed inwards. According to Tantric literatu-re, when prana is kept in the body with the help of mudras, the mind becomes introverted which leads to pratyahara – withdrawal of our senses – as well as dharana (concentration).

Mudras can be divided into five different categories:

HASTA / HAND MUDRA
These lead the energy created in our hands back into the body. You create an

energy path that flows from the brain to the hands and then back again. If you are aware of this process, an inner awareness is created quickly. Mudras in this category are: jnana mudra, chin mudra, yoni mudra, bhairava mudra, and hridayamudra.

MANA / HEAD MUDRA

These techniques are an important part of Kundalini yoga and many are used as meditation techniques. Here you use eyes, ears, nose, tongue and lips. Mudras in this category are: shambhavi mudra, nasikagra drishti, khechari mudra, khaki mudra, bhujangini mudra, bhoochari mudra, akashi mudra, shanmukhi mudra, and unmani mudra.

KAYA MUDRA

These exercises are combined with asanas, breathing techniques and concentration. Mudras in this category are: vipareeta karani mudra, pashinee mudra, prana mudra, yoga mudra, manduki mudra and tadagi mudra.

BANDHA / LOCK

These exercises combine mudras and bandhas. They charge the system with prana and prepare for the awakening of Kundalini Shakti. Techniques in this category are maha mudra, maha bheda mudra, and maha vedha mudra.

Adhara: these techniques direct the prana from the lower parts of the body to the brain. Techniques that use sexual energy belong to this group and are extremely powerful. Techniques in this category are ashwini mudra and vajroli/sahajoli mudra.

MUDRAS AND OUR ELEMENTS

In the yogic tradition, our hands are like a map of our well-being. Different points in our hands are directly linked to other body parts and our psyche. By making different mudras or hand positions, we stimulate these points and energy paths.

Our physical body, like our surroundings, is made up of five different elements: earth, water, fire, air and ether (space). Many people know the first four elements, but ether(space) is often unknown. Ether (space) is a subtle energy, celestial energy that exists high above our earth. In our body, ether is the space within us at the cellular level.

Imbalances in our elements weaken our immune system which in the long run leads to illness. These deficiencies or imbalances can be corrected by connecting different parts of the body in a specific way by mudras. Mudras create electromagnetic currents in the body, so-called energy loops. Each element is also associated with a chakra. When the element is balanced, the chakra is also affected and in turn, affects the energy (vayu) that belongs to the chakra's area.

Finger	Element/tattwa	chakra	energy/vayu
Thumb	Fire/agni	Manipura	Samana
Index finger	Air/vayu	Anahata	Prana
Middle finger	Ether/akasha	Vishuddhi	Udana
The ring finger	Earth/prithvi	Mooladhara	Apana
Little finger	Water/apas	Swadhisthana	Vyana

HASTA MUDRA PRANAYAMA
(4 four steps)

SEQUENCE
1. Chin mudra pranayama.

Sit in a comfortable meditation position. Extend the spine and neck. Place your hands, palms facing up, on your knees. Press your thumb against the index fing-er and let the other fingers point straight out. Sit still, close your eyes and follow your natural breathing for a few minutes.

Chin mudra opens up the lower lobes of the lungs and stimulates apana vayu (prana that moves down from the navel to the perineum). Physically, it is re-sponsible for the expulsion of toxins in the body.

Sit still and follow the breathing that moves in and out of the nose. Two to three minutes.

2. Chin maya mudra pranayama.

Now fold in your fingers without touching your palms. Hold your thumb against your index finger.

Chin maya mudra pranayama opens up the middle lobes of our lungs and stimulates the samana vayu (prana that moves from left to right in the area around the abdomen). Physically, it is responsible for digestion and our ability to assimilate the nutrients in our food. On a subtle level, it affects our ability to absorb (and learn from) experiences in our life.

Sit still and follow the breathing that moves in and out of the nose. Two to three minutes.

3. Aadi mudra pranayama.

Now grab the thumbs with other your fingers and place the fists on the knees with the back of the hand up.

Aadi mudra pranayama opens the upper lobes of our lungs. It stimulates the udana vayu (prana that moves upwards towards the head and outwards in our extremities). Physically, it is responsible for healing and balancing our sense organs. On a subtle level, it is responsible for balancing our perception.

Sit still and follow the breathing that moves in and out of the nose. Two to three minutes.

4. Brahma mudra pranayama.

Hold the position of the hands, but turn them so that the wrists are facing upwards and the knuckles are facing each other. Press your hands against your body level with your pelvis.

Brahma mudra pranayama opens up the whole lung. It opens up vyana vayu – the energy that makes us go on a bit longer, the last boost. It balances and starts our other pranas in the body when they become low. It revitalizes the whole system. Sit still and follow the breathing that moves in and out of the nose. Two to three minutes.

BANDHA AND GRANTHI

Traditionally, bandhas are classified as part of mudras. In Hatha Yoga Pradipika and old tantric texts, mudras and bandhas are seen as a whole, they are not separated. Bandhas are linked to mudras and to pranayamas. Bandhas are a technique that creates a unique lock in the body.

The word bandha means to hold or lock-in Sanskrit. It describes the physical effect created in the body and the retention of prana. Bandhas lock the energy into specific parts of the body and control the flow to the sushumna nadi to create a spiritual awakening.

Bandhas should be learned as a separate technique before practicing them together with mudras and pranayamas.
There are four different locking techniques: jalandhara, moola, uddiyana and

maha bandha. Maha is a combination of the first three. These three bandhas have a direct impact on our three mental points (granthis) in the body. Moola bandha is associated with Brahma granthi, uddiana bandha with Vishnu granthi, and jalandhara bandha with Rudra granthi. Granthis prevents the flow of prana along with sushumna nadi and inhibits the flow in our chakras and of Kundalini Shakti.

Brahma granthi is the first knot and is linked to Mooladhara and Swadhistana chakra. These are connected to our survival instinct and desires. When you get past the Brahma granthi, Kundalini energy gets an opportunity to wander up and past the Mooladhara and Swadhistana chakra without being drawn back by the instinctive traits of our personality.

The second knot is Vishnu granthi. It is linked to Manipura and Anahata chakra. These two chakras are connected to our emotional and mental sides. Manipura chakra controls our energy body (pranamaya kosha) and affects digestion and metabolism. Anahata controls our mental body (manomaya kosha). Together the two affect our physical body – annamaya kosha. To transcend Vishnu granthi is to no longer be bound to physical, mental and emotional desires. Relationships and energies take on a different character and meaning and are no longer limited to one's desires and needs.

The last knot is Rudra granthi, which is linked to Vishuddhi and Ajna chakra. Vishuddhi and Ajna control our body of intuition (vijnamaya kosha). When you get past the Rudra granthi, identifying with the ego stops. The experience of unmanifested consciousness appears in the Ajna and Sahasrara chakras.

"Do not search, do not seek, do not strike,
do not demand - relax.

If you relax, it will come,
if you relax, you are there.

If you relax, you start vibrating with it."

SHATKARMA

In the old Upanishads, you can read about Hatha yoga and how it is built up of shatkarmas – purification techniques. Shat means six and karma action. Shatkarmas consists of six different purification techniques. The purpose of Hatha yoga and shatkarmas is to create a balance between ida and pingala nadi, our two most important prana in the body, and thus also a balance and purity both physically and mentally.

Shatkarmas are also used to balance the three doshas: vata, pitta and kapha. According to both Hatha yoga and Ayurveda, an imbalance in the doshas causes illness. The techniques are also used before pranayamas and other more advanced yoga techniques to cleanse the body of toxins and to promote a safe and successful development purely spiritually.

Do not attempt to learn the techniques from a book. Seek instructions from a competent teacher who has adequate experience in the field.

Shatkarma includes the following different techniques:

1. NETI

A process where you clean the nasal passages. The techniques are called jala neti and sutra neti.

2. DHAUTI

A series of purification techniques are divided into three main groups: assume dhauti (internal purification), sirshadhauti (purification of the head), and hrid dhauti (purification of the neck). These techniques cleanse the entire nutrient tract from the mouth to the rectum. There are four different techniques: shankhaprakshalana and laghooshankhaprakshalana which cleanse the intestines, agnisar kriya which activates the digestive fire, kunjal where one cleanses the abdomen with the help of water, and vatsara dhauti where one cleanses the intestines with air.

3. NAULI

A method to massage and strengthen the abdominal muscles.

4. BASTI

Techniques to clean the colon.

5. KAPALBHATI

Breathing technique to clean the frontal part of the brain.

6. TRATAKA

A technique to develop the power of concentration by intensively focusing on a point or an object. According to many Tantric yogis, it is the most powerful method of obtaining siddhis (paranormal abilities).

The six shatkarmas consist of different variations of exercises. Advice and contraindications should be adhered to. During pregnancy, only jala neti (nasal rinsing) and trataka are recommended. While Shatkarmas are cleansing and invigorating, they are not the main purpose of the techniques. Shatkarmas are done to promote the health of those who practice yoga and to awaken and direct the energies in the body and mind safely so they do not flow the wrong way. People suffering from any medical illness should consult a competent teacher before doing any of the exercises.

JALA NETI / NOSE RINSE

Jala neti is a purification technique that all yogis practice before each yoga session. Jala neti cleanses the nasal passages and sinuses from mucus and contaminants. The air can then flow freely through the nose. It counteracts illnesses of the respiratory tract and promotes healthy ears, eyes and throat. Tensions in the face are released. It has a calming effect on the brain. Anxiety, anger and depression are relieved. Jala neti stimulates nerve endings in the nose and promotes the sense of smell. A balance is created between the right and left nostrils as well as the right and left side of the brain. This, in turn, creates a balance and harmony between the body and the mind. The most important thing is that jala neti helps awaken Ajna chakra.

"WHO AM I?

AM I MY BODY, OR CAN I EXPERIENCE IT?

AM I MY THOUGHTS, OR DO I HEAR THEM?

AM I MY FEELINGS, OR DO I FEEL THEM?

AM I MY INTUITION, OR DO I SENSE IT?

WHO AM I, I CANNOT BE TWO?

I AM THE BEING, THE CONSCIOUSNESS,
THE ONE WHO EXPERIENCES EVERYTHING.
IN MYSELF BUT ALSO AROUND

I'M THAT, IT'S ME. OM TAT TVASI"

LESSON NO. 2

YOGA NIDRA DO YOU LEARN IN MODULE 3. THINGS TO THINK BEFORE LEADING CLASS – SEE MODULE NO.1.

LONG SHAVASANA – DEAD MAN'S POSTURE/RELAXATION.

PRANAYAMA – YOGIC BREATHING.

SUPTA PAWANMUKTASANA – LEG LOCK.

MARJARIASANA – THE CAT.

NAUKA SANCHALANA – ROWING THE BOAT.

PASCHIMOTTANASANA – THE PLIERS.

MATSYASANA – THE FISH.

SHAVASANA – DEAD MAN'S POSTURE.

SHAVA UDARAKARSHANASANA – THE UNIVERSAL POSITION.

SHAVASANA – DEAD MAN'S POSTURE.

BHUJANGASANA – THE COBRA.

SHASHANKASANA – THE HARE.

SHAVASANA – DEAD MAN'S POSTURE.

YOGA NIDRA – DEEP RELAXATION.

END WITH – HARI OM TAT SAT, 3 TIMES.

THEN – OM SRI DURGAYAI NAMAH, 1 TIME.

INSTRUCTIONS FOR ASANAS LESSON NO. 2.

LONG SHAVASANA – DEAD MAN´S POSTURE/RELAXATION.

Execution: *See module 1.*

PRANAYAMA – YOGIC BREATHING.

Execution: Place one hand on the stomach and one hand on the chest to begin with. Inhale, fill your stomach like a balloon, then fill your chest - at the front, under your arms and into the back, hold your breath at the collarbones (use the chin to hold your breath), then release your breath - first from your chest and then your stomach. Empty your lungs (bahir kumbhaka) and then start again. 5-10 min.

SUPTA PAWANMUKTASANA – LEG LOCK.

Execution: Lie on your back with your legs touching and your arms alongside your body. Inhale and lift the right leg, exhale, bend the leg, clasp your hands around the knee and pull the leg towards the upper body. On one exhale, lift your head up and bring your chin up towards your knee. Press the left leg into the mat. Stay and breathe. Exhale and bring your head down, inhale, stretch out your right leg, exhale and bring your leg down. Do the same with the left leg. 2-3 min.

MARJARIASANA – THE CAT.

Execution: Kneel on all fours. Place your hands directly underneath your shoulders and your knees directly underneath your hips. Keep your back and neck straight and look down at the floor. Exhale, arch your back. Inhale, return to the starting position.. 2-3 min.

NAUKA SANCHALANA – ROWING THE BOAT.

Execution: Sit with straight legs and grab your thumbs. Inhale - clench your fists as if they were holding oars, exhale and extend your hands towards your feet. Keep your knees soft in the extended position so that your lumbar spine is protected. 2-3 min.

PASCHIMOTTANASANA – THE PLIERS.

Execution: Sit with both legs straight out in front of you, preferably on the edge of a folded blanket so that your pelvis tilts slightly forward. Inhale, stretch your back and fold forward with your back straight as you exhale. Push your chest forward. Wrap the index finger and middle finger around the big toe and create a lock with the thumbs. Then inhale and roll up. Remember to keep your legs slightly bent. 2-3 min.

MATSYASANA – THE FISH.

Execution: Lie on your back. Place your hands under your buttocks with your palms facing up. Raise as high as you can on your elbows and look down at your feet. Then tilt your head back and push your chest up. Try to let the scalp rest against the floor. Keep your feet together. 2-3 min.

SHAVASANA – DEAD MAN'S POSTURE.

Execution: Move the legs apart, let your feet fall to the sides and lie with the arms slightly away from the body. Turn your palms upwards. Stretch your spine, tip your chin down and breathe deeply with your stomach. Concentrate on your breathing and feel the whole body from the inside out to completely relax. 2-3 min.

SHAVA UDARAKARSHANASANA – THE UNIVERSAL POSITION.

Execution: Lie on your back, lift your right leg and bend at the knee. Place the left hand on the right knee, exhale and pull the knee over to the left side. Extend your right arm out at a 90-degree angle to your body and turn your head to look at your right hand. Try to push the right shoulder blade into the mat. Stay here and breathe in and out. Inhale and roll back onto your back. Repeat on the left side. 2-3 min. on each side.

BHUJANGASANA – THE COBRA.

Execution: Lie on your stomach with your arms bent and palms flat on the floor underneath your shoulders. Inhale and bring your head and chest up high. Keep your feet together. Place your hands on your chest and then push yourself up a few inches without pulling your shoulders up. 2-3 min.

SHASHANKASANA – THE HARE.

Execution: This pose is recommended after backbends. Lie on your stomach, put your hands under your shoulders and push yourself back so you sit on your heels, lean forward with your forehead touching the floor and stretch your arms out in front. Stay here and breathe in and out. Become aware of your breathing. 2-3 min.

MOOLADHARA CHAKRA (READ ABOUT THE CHAKRANA IN MODUL 4)

To practice regularly for a month.

Chakra and kshetram localization/activation and purification by moola bandha, contraction of the abdomen, first slowly. Breathe in – hold the breath

… feel the pulsation a few centimeters up from the diaphragm inside the body and pronounce the mantra Lam in time with the pulse beat and then release the lock … then quickly and with Lam in step with breathing. Then sit for about five minutes with a powerful moola bandha and feel the pulsation of the chakra and chanta Lam in time. You can also visualize the color and yantra.

Nasikagra drishti – focus on the tip of the nose without closing your eyes. If your eyes get tired during this exercise, you can close them for a moment and then return to the exercise.

KNOWLEDGE TEST MODULE 2

ANSWER AS FULLY AS YOU CAN, THEN CHECK IF YOU ANSWERED CORRECTLY. PRACTICE UNTIL YOU KNOW THE ANSWERS BY HEART.

1. WHAT ARE OUR FIVE BODIES?

2. EXPLAIN WHAT OUR FIVE PRANA VAYUS ARE.

3. DESCRIBE THE ASANAS.

4. DESCRIBE THE PRANAYAMAS.

5. DESCRIBE THE MUDRAS.

6. DESCRIBE THE BANDHAS AND GRANTHIS.

7. DESCRIBE SHATKARMA.

8. WHY IS IT SO IMPORTANT TO RINSE YOUR NOSE BEFORE YOGA?

9. DESCRIBE MOOLADHARA CHAKRA, ITS ELEMENT, YANTRA, COLOR, NUMBER OF PETALS AND ATTRIBUTES.

10. RELATE SOME POWERFUL EXERCISES TO ACTIVATE, CLEAN AND BALANCE MOOLADHARA CHAKRA.

MODULE 3

RAJA YOGA, YOGA SUTRAS AND MEDITATION. WE STUDY YOGA PHILOSOPHY AND LEARN TO LEAD YOGA NIDRA AND AJAPA JAPA

We study Raja yoga and yoga philosophy by reading the most important sutras from Patanjali's classic work, 'Yoga Sutras'. We learn to lead the meditation ajapa japa and the deep relaxation yoga nidra, both from the tantric tradition. We study the Swadhisthana chakra and practice our exercises to cleanse, balance and activate the chakra. We continue to practice the role of yoga teacher with lesson no. 3 of 8.

Knowledge test: Answer the questions related to module 3. Practice lesson no. 3 with at least 1 participant and humbly accept feedback from them. Ask questions afterward – how was the pace, did you keep to time, did you speak loudly enough, and how well did you understand the exercises?

RAJA YOGA

SHIVA AND SHAKTI. YOGA PHILOSOPHY'S TWO PRINCIPLES – CONSCIOUSNESS AND ENERGY, MAN & WOMAN

CLASSICAL YOGA & ITS PHILOSOPHY

In classical yoga and its yoga philosophy, Prakriti (Shakti) is described as cosmic energy. It is the original essence behind everything we can experience, both rough and subtle. Prakriti is not in solid form, there is nothing that can be "touched". Prakriti acts as a tool for Purusha (Shiva). Our mind is a result of Prakriti. For consciousness to be able to experience and expand and experience itself, Prakriti is needed. Without Prakriti, consciousness cannot become self-aware.

The qualities of prakritis are what build up our bodies and our world. It carries karma and coexists through which living beings come into existence and which also shapes our senses.

Prakriti consists of three qualities – sattva, rajas and tamas. These three qualities are a basis for the other elements.

PRAKRITI	**PURUSHA**
All experiences.	*The experience.*
Manifested.	*Unmanifest.*
Background to everything.	*Eternal subject.*
Materially and mentally.	*Infinite amount.*

THREE PRINCIPLES BUILD A COSMOS

It is thus from these three principles that our whole world is built – in varying combinations, rajas, tamas and sattva. The cosmos, society and every human being are governed by the interactions between these gunas.

There are two basic "laws" that describe how the interaction between these three works. The first is the "law of alternation" and by that is meant that they are in constant motion and collaboration with each other. In sattva, rajas and tamas also exist. In rajas, tamas and sattva exist and in tamas rajas and sattva exist. They work together all the time.

The second is the "law of continuity". By this, it means that when a guna has become dominant, it tends to be so for some time to come.

In yoga, a sattvic state is seen as something of a higher quality, the state that causes us to develop spiritually. Yoga practice consists of two steps. To develop a sattvic condition and to then go beyond this condition. This means that we should first purify the body and mind and then go beyond the body and mind and experience what is our true nature beyond all manifestation. There is also a hidden, mysterious knowledge tradition about activating our chakra system that we will go through later. The basic pre-condition for the chakra system to be activated is that the sushumna is open, and that is only when you are in a sattvic state. In scientific terms, these three gunas are described as:

SATTVA
Pure vibration / balanced.

RAJAS
Movement.

TAMAS
Inertia / slow / immobility.

One talks about three human characters. The guna that dominates us determines what character we have. You should know the different personality traits and adapt the yoga practice accordingly.

If you are tamasic or slow, it is good with a dynamic form of yoga where you get the activity going in the body and in this way can create balance. Hatha yoga or physical work suits tamasic people.

If you are rajasic or mobile, you often have difficulty concentrating. Here it is important to have a lot of relaxation but to be able to relax and release tension, a dynamic form of yoga is required here as well. You exhaust your body and mind to then be able to relax more easily. Hatha yoga, Bhakti yoga (e.g. kirtan), Japa yoga and Karma yoga are suitable for rajasic people.

If you are sattvic or balanced, it is already easy to focus and concentrate and then it is well suited to satsang and studies. But even if you are sattvic, you need to work with the body. This is to create balance in the already balanced thought activity.

A rule to follow is that inertia is balanced with movement, and movement is balanced with even more movement. We always start with the outer, the surface, our body and go inward, deeper...balance and activate. We always start with the movement. Always.

ISHVARA

Yoga is a practical method based on the samkhya philosophy, but unlike samkhya, yoga's view of creation is theistic.

In classical yoga, the god or creator is called Ishvara in Sanskrit. Ishvara is said to be the force that creates, maintains and destroys the world through the three forms Brahma, Vishnu and Shiva, as well as their female counterparts Saraswati, Lakshmi and Kali.

Although Ishvara is very similar to our Western god, they differ in that Ishvara works through different gods and goddesses, it has different shapes and manifestations. Ishavara can also be worshiped in a female form and is then called Ishvari. This is common in many yoga traditions and especially those of tantric origin. Ishvari is then equated with Shakti.

Ishvara is not described separately in samkhya, but in many yoga traditions, Ishvara is described as Purusha (Shiva in tantrism).

DARSHANS

Vedas are writings composed of rishis (sight/medium) and yogis about 5000 years ago (they can also be much older). These describe the wisdom behind the cosmic mind, which is said to be the origin of the universe and creation. These writings have from the beginning been passed on orally and then written down. Yoga has its roots in Vedic teachings. Rishis gave Vedic knowledge a practical form, yoga.

From the Vedas, six philosophical paths/views were developed, shad darshans, which means "six ways of seeing" or "six ways of insight". Classical yoga as described by Patanjali in the Yoga Sutras is one of these.

Hiranyagarbha, the sun god and the cosmic creator is traditionally said to be the creator of the yoga system.

The six Vedic / spiritual paths:

1. Nyaya – logical doctrine – Gautama.
2. Vaisheshika – atomic doctrine – Kannada.
3. Samkhya – the doctrine of the cosmic principle – Kapila.
4. Yoga – the doctrine of yoga – Hiranyagarbha.
5. Purva Mimamsa / vedanta – ritual doctrine – Jasmine.
6. Yttara Mimamsa / Vedanta – theological doctrine – badarayana.

Nayaya and vaisheshka are teachings based on logical philosophy. These can be compared to Plato's philosophy as we know it in the West.

Samkhya is the philosophy behind yoga and ayurveda. It is based on a scientific approach that explores both our inner and outer reality. Samkhya describes tattwas / cosmic principles that one tries to gain insight into and experience with the help of various yogic exercises. Samkhya describes the knowledge behind the different elements and yoga is a technique that should purify and balance the corresponding elements in ourselves.

Purva Mimamsa refers to Karma yoga where it acts as a channel for the creative energy of the universe. You work and contribute with selfless services/work to people and society. It is also part of focusing on a prayer or a mantra during the work. This cleanses both the mind and the body and is a good preparation for meditation.

Uttara Mimamsa is the system where you go in-depth for the Vedic texts. One discusses god, the soul, the absolute and their interaction with each other.

AUM

A common symbol in yoga is Om. The symbol is made up of three syllables that together form a whole. In Sanskrit, the vowel "o" consists of "a + u". So Om can also be spelled as Aum. It represents the trinity of our existence.

The symbol A-u-m consists of three "curves", a semicircle and a point. The largest "curve" that is also at the bottom refers to our waking state when our consciousness is turned outwards and when we take in the environment with the help of our sense organs. It's called jagarat. That it is symbolized by the largest "curve" because it is the most common state we are in. Beta waves dominate in this state – we are aware.

The second largest curve which is at the top of the symbol refers to deep sleep and our unconscious state. We neither dream nor feel desire. This condition is called sushputi. Delta waves dominate in this state – we are unconscious.

The smallest curve that is between these two refers to our dream state, swapana. Here the consciousness is turned inwards, you experience the world with closed eyes. Theta waves dominate in this state. The experience of the subconscious.

The point in the symbol refers to our fourth state of consciousness which in Sanskrit is called turiya. Here we look neither outwards nor inwards but are in pure being. That is the unmanifest, state of Purusha. Alpha waves dominate in this state – we are superconscious.

The semicircle refers to the Maya, which separates the point turiya from the "three curves". Maya symbolizes what hinders our ability to experience our true nature. That the semicircle is just half, tells us that Maya cannot change the true experience that exists within us, the stillness/being/bliss. Maya can only decide what is manifested.

Aum thus symbolizes the manifested and the unmanifested. What we can see and what we cannot see and represent the trinity of our existence. The sound and vibrations that occur when we sound Om / Aum affect our whole being on all these levels and are a very strong mantra. It permeates our entire interior and makes us vibrate in step with the universe. Aum – the sound/vibration of the universe and creation.

VIVEKA

Patanjali (the author of the Yoga Sutras) describes something called viveka, ie. discernment. The purpose of eight-step yoga (classical yoga) is precisely to develop viveka within us, ie. awareness, which is a prerequisite for understanding the purpose of yoga.

It requires a sharp ability to pay attention and be able to distinguish the expe-

riencer from the experience, see what is our true identity and what is perishable. We also need sharp attention to see what is the reason for our ignorance of this – ie. to miss what is changeable for immutable, to miss what is destructive for edification, to miss desires for need, to identify with the ego instead of the true self.

VAIRAGYA

When we have developed viveka, a change takes place in us. We begin to let go of our desires. This is called vairagya. We no longer cling to what will disappear anyway. When we understand the principle of transience, we can take a more understanding approach to life's worries and troubles. If you read about the yoga philosophy, you understand that Buddha was enlightened in India and was about the same time as Patanjali and where he took his inspiration for the eight-fold path. People often talk about Buddhism as a cousin of the yoga philosophy. Many of the ideas are similar.

RAGA

Everything that we experience and "take in" from our surroundings happens with our senses. Through our eyes (sight), ears (hearing), nose (scent), tongue (taste), body/skin (feeling), and mind (thoughts, feelings, images). They can then be divided into comfortable, uncomfortable and neutral experiences. Most often we want to re-experience the comfortable experiences and provide enjoyment. We want to recreate these experiences time and time again. This is called raga.

Events that we experience as painful and unpleasant, we want to avoid. Most of our time we try to find what gives us pleasure and avoid what is painful. This creates dissatisfaction and a divided mind. We do not feel satisfied with what is. We do not accept life for what it is.

DRASHTA BHAVA

In yoga, we try to create a third approach called drashta bhava. This can be translated as "witness attitude". Here we try to have a neutral and relaxed attitude to our thoughts, both negative and positive. This approach together with viveka leads to liberation, the ultimate purpose of yoga. To be free from desire, not to be controlled by thoughts and feelings. To be happy with what is – right now, whatever it looks like. To accept what we cannot change.

CURRENT CLASSICAL YOGA:

SATYANANDA YOGA

Today, classical yoga is taught through, among other things, Satyananda yoga. It is a system developed by Swami Satyananda Saraswati. Here they use ancient and traditional techniques. Asanas to create balance between body and mind, pranayamas to work with the energy body and meditation to calm and focus the mind. Tradition also teaches the yogic lifestyle in general to both the "ordinary modern man" and the more devoted practitioner. Everyone can take part in yoga. Jnana, Bhakti and Karma yoga, among others, are also part of the Satyanada system.

In Satyananda yoga, one takes into account the whole being of man, not just the body. You want to give the individual an opportunity to discover and develop all aspects of one's personality with the help of yoga. It is believed that change is something that happens with regular practice, under full presence and awareness. Not by pushing the body or mind beyond its means.

SRI SWAMI SIVANANDA SARASWATI

Swami Satyananda's guru and perhaps India's most famous yoga personality – Sri Swami Sivananda Saraswati, was born in Pattamadai, in 1887. Sivananda worked as a doctor before giving up his job to find his guru in the Himalayas. He settled in Rishikesh where he was initiated into dashnami sannyasa by his guru Swami Vishwananda Saraswati in 1924. Over the years, he and his disciples wrote hundreds of books and articles on yoga and spirituality to spread the knowledge to the general public. Sri Swami Sivananda wanted to give the needy the knowledge that could help them, whether it was about improving physical health, creating peace of mind or developing spiritually. This still characterizes Satyananda yoga today.

SWAMI SATYANANDA SARASWATI

Swami Satyananda Saraswati was born in Almora in 1923. At the age of nineteen, he met Sukhman Giri, from Juna-Akhara, a Tantric yogini from Nepal. From her, he learned, among other things, the tantric nyasa techniques, which he developed further with Swami Sivananda. Nyasa is a technique for raising awareness by placing different energies in the body parts. From there, he then developed the world-famous deep relaxation yoga nidra. In 1943 he then met his guru Swami Sivananda and was initiated into dashnami sannyasa in 1947. After serving his guru's mission for twelve years, Satyanada began his journey through India as an ascetic to discover the needs of society. In 1956, Swami Satyananda founded the International Yoga Fellowship and in 1963 the Bihar School Of Yoga, hoping to spread ancient yogic knowledge to all corners of the world. For twenty years, Swami Satyananda then traveled around the world, spreading the knowledge of yoga. He and his disciples also authored over eighty books on yoga, tantra, and spirituality. In 1984, he founded the "Yoga Research Foundation" and "Sivananda Math" to help those who were disadvantaged in society.

YOGA FORMS

In Satyananda yoga, the following forms of yoga are applied:

JNANA YOGA

The path of spiritual insight is where one, through intellectual and theoretical knowledge, studies life and tries to distinguish the true from the perishable. This path is suitable for theoretically inclined people.

BHAKTI YOGA

The path of devotion and love consists of song and dance or meditation on an image of a guru or the divine. The practicer strives to create a personal relationship with the divine and merge with it.

KARMA YOGA

Selfless service is where you help other people and society without taking advantage of it or shining in the glory.

HATHA YOGA

Here you want to balance and strengthen the physical and mental body as a preparation for the more advanced exercises in kundalini yoga. Asanas, pranayamas, bandhas and shatkarmas are used.

RAJA YOGA – CLASSIC YOGA

The path of meditation. This refers to the system described in Patanjali's Yoga Sutras.

KRIYA YOGA

Satyananda taught Kriya yoga based on the secret exercises of yoga and tantra shastras. Kriya means "activity" or "movement" and refers to the natural movement of consciousness. Kriya yoga does not stop the movements of the mind but instead creates an activity in the mind that leads to a conscious increase and awakening. There are seventy kriyas of which twenty are best known and used.

THE TRADITIONS

In addition to the yogic tradition, Satyananda yoga also includes the Tantric and Vedic traditions.

Tantra refers to practical exercises, which lead to the expansion of the human consciousness and the awakening of Kundalini Shakti. The principle behind the tantric system is that one uses the material world and experiences of it to become enlightened.

Tantra is often described as a sexual tradition where you want to enhance the sexual experience. Originally, tantra was intended to awaken Kundalini Shakti, which is a dormant potential force in man.

There are many tantric paths and the common denominator of these paths is the use of mantras, yantras (concentration symbols used to liberate consciousness), chakras, mandalas (discovering macrocosm in microcosm), tapasya (self-purification), Raja yoga, pranayama, shaktipat (power transmission) and tantric initiations to reach awakening.

Tantrism advocates a life in which the qualities of the intellect and the heart are exploited. To be able to discern and focus with the help of the intellect and to be able to see and experience with the heart the unseen, the cosmic consciousness beyond the material.

The Vedic tradition is one of the oldest preserved spiritual traditions in existence. It advocates the divine as the ultimate truth and life accordingly in the material world.

Central to Vedic doctrine is that God is constantly present, omniscient and omnipotent while the individual is only an actor. To experience the reality that is satyam (truth), shivam (favorable) and sundaram (beautiful), the individual should live a life where one strives to harmonize thoughts, behavior and actions. A meditative contemplation, belief in God and oneself. Living in harmony with, and being grateful for, the environment and nature and experiencing unity are the foundations of the Vedic tradition.

All the Vedic and Tantric traditions are held together by yoga. Yoga is the practical principle of the spiritual paths that leads to increased awareness and self-insight.

RAJA YOGA – THE ROYAL PATH

Patanjali never gave his system any specific title. He simply called it yoga. In time, however, his method became known as Patanjali's yoga and or classical yoga. Patanjali's yoga is one of the different forms of Raja yoga (Raja means royal):

Kundalini yoga (also called Laya yoga).

Kriya yoga.

Yoga mantra.

Dhyana yoga.

Patanjali yoga.

Raja yoga is the doctrine of the mind. Here you explore your inner world to be able to take advantage of the strength and knowledge that we have. Raja yoga teaches different methods to create a focused mind. It is based on mental discipline.

Patanjali himself defined his method as "elimination of mental fluctuations" – Yoga chitta vritti nirodha. Usually translated to – when the mind is still, yoga occurs. The mind can be described as the visible part of the pure consciousness and divided into the conscious, the subconscious and the unconscious. Patanjali's definition means that "yoga is the control of the pattern of consciousness".

VIYOGA

Who is experiencing this?

Most people know that yoga means union, but in the Yoga Sutras, Patanjali describes yoga as a process of separation. This can be explained by the Samkhya philosophy, which is the foundation of the Yoga Sutras.

Samkhya divides existence and individuality into two different aspects that we have touched on before – Purusha and Prakriti. The existence and the individual are created when these two merge. Purusha refers to the one who sees / experiences, drashta. Prakriti refers to the seen, drishya.

Practicing yoga and its process leads to viyoga, which is a separation between the one who experiences and the seen. This in turn leads to yoga, the association that is the very development of yoga, the culmination. At first Purusha and

Prakriti must be separated from each other and then it is understood that these are the same.

It can also be described that the pure consciousness (Purusha) is broken down by incorrect identification with mind and body (Prakriti). The purpose of yoga is to release pure consciousness from the mind and body.

The experience of the difference and separation between Purusha and Prakriti leads to the realization that everything is the same.

"A method by which consciousness is disconnected from entanglement with mind and the manifested world. Yoga (union) is the result"

EIGHT STEPS / ASHTANGA

Patanjali describes a series of techniques that have a slow and harmonizing effect on our minds and perception. The most important thing in Patanjali's system is described in the eight steps. The first five steps are preparatory to the other three steps and belong to bhairanga / outer yoga. Ashtanga means eight different steps and should not be confused in this context with the modern Ashtanga yoga developed by yoga master Shri K. Pattabhi Jois.

You must not see the first five steps as a staircase, you can also see it as a wheel where by working with one step you also influence the others.

1. Yama – is about moral discipline in social life.

2. Niyama – is about restraint on a personal level.

3. Asana – sitting position/body position. This refers to the correct meditation position/lotus position so that you can remain immobile during the meditation and are not distracted by the physical body.

"I'M WAITING TO LEAVE THIS BODY, BUT I'M NOT GOING TO LEAVE IT UNTIL I GET MY RETURN TICKET. I DO NOT WANT EMANCIPATION, MOKSHA, OR ANY PERSONAL SATISFACTION WHICH COMES WITH SPIRITUAL ENLIGHTENMENT. MY AIM AND ASPIRATION IN THIS AND ALL FUTURE LIVES IS TO HELP OTHERS. TO WIPE THE TEARS OF SUFFERING AND PAIN FROM THE EYES OF EVERY PERSON WHO IS SEEKING SOLACE, PEACE, PLENTY AND PROSPERITY. THAT IS THE ONLY PURPOSE OF MY LIFE"

(SWAMI SATYANANDA SARASWATI)

4. Pranayama – respiratory regulation / control of prana / kumbhaka. By controlling breathing, you can control the life force/prana in the body and calm the mind.

5. Pratyahara – removal of sensory impressions. By blocking sensory impressions, one is not distracted by the external environment.

The last three steps belong to antharanga / inner yoga. To develop in-depth and succeed with these steps, one must have absorbed the first five preparatory steps. The steps before pratyahara gradually dissolve external obstacles that one has in life while the exercises after eliminate thoughts and inner images so that the mind is still. Ida (our inner world) becomes balanced with pingala (our outer world) so that the sushumna (our supersensible world) begins to exist during samadhi.

6. Dharana – concentration. Focus on a meditation object.

7. Dhyana – meditation. After a longer concentration, you naturally sink into meditation. Here one is fulfilled by the meditation object.

8. Samadhi – liberation/ecstasy / superconscious. Meditation eventually leads to samadhi. Here the movements of the mind have stopped and you become one with the meditation object and experience powerful ecstasy/joy. There are twelve stages of samadhi and the last stage leads to the liberation of the cycle of rebirths.

The eight steps gradually balance our five koshas (shells): annamaya, pranamaya, manomaya, vijnamaya and anandamaya. The boundary between the shells is loosened from the coarsest – the body, annamaya kosha, to the most subtle, our innermost interior – anandamaya kosha.

YAMA

Satya – truth, to be true to oneself and others.

Ahimsa – do not be involved in the killing.

Asteya – do not steal, not take more than you need and share.

Aparighara – not to be greedy, to live materially simply.

Brahmacharya – chastity. To live ascetically, not indulge in pleasures as they are considered to distract one from reaching the goal of yoga.

NIYAMA

Saucha – purity of speech and action, sensory impressions (media, television, radio), food, hygiene.

Santosha – contentment, to be happy with what you have. If we focus on what we do not have, we create even more emptiness within ourselves. If we focus on shortages, we get even more shortages (the law of attraction).

Tapas – self-discipline, hardening of the inner fire.

Swadhyaya – studies.

Ishwara pranidhara – to surrender one's will to the higher will.

Yamas thus create a balance in our interaction with the outside world and niyamas harmonize our inner feelings. These rules are created to balance our external actions with our internal settings. The mind affects our external actions at the same time as our external actions affect the mind. If our actions are not good, the mind will also be negatively affected, which creates a vicious circle as a distracted mind creates less good actions. Yamas and niyamas are designed to break the vicious circle. It can be difficult to follow these rules in full, but even a small change does a lot to balance the mind.

PATANJALIS YOGA SUTRAS

Patanjali's work consists of one hundred and ninety-six sutras. The word sutra itself is often incorrectly translated as verse. The actual translation is "to thread in a row", which also describes how the sutras are linked to each other and carry an underlying continuity. The work is seen as the most accurate and scientific yogic text ever written down.

Who Patanjali was and when he lived is still unclear. It has also not been possible to determine when his work was written and whether he was a man or a woman. There is still some evidence that he must have lived about 300-400 years BC.

Patanjali gives us a range of techniques that gradually balance and harmonize our minds. The unique thing is that Patanjali does not describe a single yoga position in the way we are usually used to. Here, instead, the focus is on yoga from a moral perspective. When Patanjali talked about asana, he referred to a steady and comfortable position to sit and meditate in.

Many great masters and yogis have translated and interpreted Patanjali's work.

The following sutras are some of the most important to know:

3:2

Cause of suffering.

Avidyāsmitārāgadveṣābhiniveśāh kleśāh

Avidy: erroneous knowledge, asmit: I-experience, raga: liking, dves: reluctance, abhiniveh: fear of death, klesah: suffering.

Klesha is the suffering that is present in everyone. The basis of all suffering accor-

ding to Patanjali is incorrect identification with the experience. Everyone carries a subconscious suffering but we are seldom aware of it in our daily life, all the musts and chores block the experience of it.

We rarely become aware of our fear of dying, even if it is in our subconscious. The fear of dying is the basis of our greatest suffering. Kleshas is like a chain of misfortune that begins with our ignorance of our true nature based on our ego. We try to find pleasure and avoid suffering, which in turn creates fear and tension. The solution to being free from suffering is meditation.

4:2

The root cause.

Avidyākṣetramuttareṣām prasuptatanuvichchhinnodārāṇām

Avidya: incorrect knowledge, ksetram: area, uttaresam: of the following, prasupta: dormant, tanu: weak, vichchhinna: alternating, udaranam: fully active.

Avidya is the field of dormant, weak, alternating and fully active states of kleshas.

Avidya is the basis of the other four kleshas: asmita, raga, dweshta and abhinivesha. These are either dormant, weak, alternating or fully active. When we learn to deal with avidya, we can also more easily learn to deal with the other four kleshas. Avidya is about the ignorance of our true nature. To find our way back to our true nature, we must learn to control the kleshas.

5:2

Incorrect knowledge.

Anityāśuchiduhkhānātmasu nityaśuchisukhātmakhyātiravidyā

Anitya: not eternal, asuchi: unclean, duhkha: pain, natmasu: not atman, nitya: eternal, suchi: pure, sukha: goodness, atma: self, khyati: knowledge, avidya: erroneous knowledge.

Avidya means that one confuses the eternal, impure and evil with the eternal, pure, good and atman.

Avidaya is about ignorance of our true nature and our identification with the body. We are free from Avidaya by developing our discernment, viveka. Through viveka we can distinguish between our body and atman, our inner true self.

Avidaya is also called Maya. In a cosmic context, it is called maya and on an individual level, it is called avidaya.

6:2
Separation, I, ego.
Dṛgdarśanaśaktyorekātmatevāsmitā

Drg: Purusha, the power of consciousness, darsana: the seen, saktyoh: of the two forces, ekatmate: identity, eva: like that, dodge: I-feeling.

Asmita can be described as an identification of Purusha as a Buddhi. Asmita means that our inner consciousness, our true self is mixed with our existence, body, actions and mind. When our true self is expressed through the body, actions and mind, it is called asmita. Purusha is identified by its means of expression/instrument.

This can be expressed in different ways. As identification with the body or in a more intellectually developed person as identification with the more developed sensory functions.

Our ability to see, think and hear comes from Purusha, which is expressed through our senses. When we mix these it is called asmita.

It is Shakti, the power of Purusha that lies behind the ability to think, see, etc. which is mixed with the actual means/instrument with which these are expressed.

By meditating, we can realize that Purusha is not a part of the body or the intellect (Buddhi). We come across asmita.

7:2

Attraction, I want.

Sukhānuśayå rāgah

Sukha: satisfaction, anusayl: accompanying, ragah: pleasure, liking.

Raga is the pleasure created by satisfaction.

Raga is about the mind constantly wanting to recreate a previous experience of pleasure.

8:2

Repulsion, I do not want.

Duhkahānuśayå dveṣah

Duhka: pain, anusayl: accompanying, dvesah: reluctance.

Dwesha is our reluctance to experience pain.

Dwesha is the opposite of raga. You want to avoid what creates discomfort. Raga and dwesha keep us in the lower stages of consciousness. As long as raga and dwesha are allowed to rule over us, we do not develop spiritually.

To like something also means that you do not like the opposite of what you like. So raga and dwesha are not opposites but two sides of the mind. Dwesha is what affects us most negatively because it is based on a lot of hatred. The elimination of dweshta allows for deeper meditation and the natural elimination of raga.

9:2

Fear of dying.

Svarasavāhī viduṣo ʹpi tathārūdho ʹbhiniveśah

Svarasavahi: persistence of self, vidusah: of the learned, api: also, tatha: like it, rudhah: dominant, abhinivesah: fear of death.

Abnivecha is the hope of being able to live and be maintained by one's power even among scholars.

This is the most dominant klesha. Fear of dying is experienced by all individuals. It is an innate inherent force that exists naturally in us, self-preservation drive. As children, we do not experience this in the same way, but the older we get, the more aware we become of it.

In those who have developed viveka, abhinivecha is almost eliminated, but in most people, it can be seen in its most active form, which can also lead to fear and panic in, for example, a serious illness. In ancient Indian texts, one can read about the cause of abhnivecha which is said to be the identification with the body.

11:2
Meditation – the solution to the elimination of kleshas.
Dhyānaheyāstadvṛttayah
Dhyana: meditation, heyah: reduces, tadvrttayah: modification, change.

The modification of the kleshas can be reduced through meditation.

We can learn to understand our fears/kleshas by observing the mind. These exist in our subconscious as well as in our conscious mind to varying degrees. In our normal daily state, we rarely see the character of the kleshas. We can not eliminate the kleshas with the help of the intellect, it can only be done with the help of meditation.

It takes a sharp ability to pay attention to become aware of how kleshas look in ourselves. For example, we may believe that we are not afraid of death even though we unconsciously are. We do not see it. Even individuals who have been engaged in spiritual development for a long time - who for several years have experienced peace and thought they are free from samskaras and kleshas, can suddenly experience obstacles and failure. The seed, root and cause of the kleshas remain and come up to the surface.

To get rid of kleshas in-depth, you need to practice the whole system of yoga. Yamas, niyamas and Kriya yoga.

By dhyana ie. to observe what happens to us mentally. This is done by paying attention to our thoughts, both good and bad, and by letting them come to the surface. In the long run, it prevents kleshas from manifesting in the most active form, which creates suffering and fear in our daily lives. In this case, one does not refer to "object focus" when talking about dhyana but assumes mouna ie. that one focuses on how kleshas look and its character and strength.

By focusing and observing, vrittis is weakened. This is the explanation for why meditation has such a calming effect on us. During meditation, our unconscious fears can come to the surface so that we become aware of them. Tensions caused by our fears/kleshas are weakened and we can relax. A feeling of inner harmony arises.

When our fears/kleshas have taken on a more latent form, we should, through our discernment / viveka, try to find the cause of the fear. Maybe you are dependent on something or maybe you want to be successful.

Dhyana (Raja yoga) and viveka (Jnana yoga) are thus two important tools in the elimination of our fears/kleshas. To prevent being drawn back to the unconscious state again – when one experiences risk becoming too difficult to deal with, Karma yoga and Bhakti yoga can be very helpful.

2:1

What is yoga?

Yogaschitta vṛitti nirodhah

Yogah: yoga, chitta: consciousness, vritti: patterns, movements, nirodhah: blocked – still.

When the movements of the mind are still, yoga occurs.

The term chitta refers to the mind, the individual consciousness on the conscious, unconscious and subconscious planes.

Nirodhah aims to block the movements of the mind, the pattern of consciousness, not the mind or consciousness itself.

This happens automatically when we sleep. The normal flow of vrittis is stopped and we are moved to another state of consciousness. We experience other things, people, events and places. With this, we can understand that within us there is something that exists independently of our body, mind and life energy/prana, something that is something completely different than any of these. This "something" is consciousness, a constant and uninterrupted state of consciousness.

Vritti can be translated as "circular" and this describes what chita's movements look like. They are like rings on the water.

So, what is yoga? Yoga is to calm the movements of the mind on all planes of consciousness. It is not about shutting down or trying to shield oneself from the external impressions that we encounter every day. What we want is to get past the experiences and visions that our consciousness creates during deep meditation and higher stages of samadhi. When this happens, yoga occurs. This is a prerequisite for the development of human consciousness.

When one ceases to identify with Prakriti, the three gunas develop our conscio-usness.

They talk about the five different characters of the mind. If you compare these with the Kundalini awakening, you can see that moodha / the sluggish mind is associated with the Mooladhara chakra where the individual consciousness is dormant.

After a period of practicing specific exercises, the consciousness is stimulated so that it directs itself to the area around the navel, the Manipura chakra. This state of consciousness is called kshipta and belongs to rajas. Most often, however, it sinks to Mooladhara chakra again and then rises to Swadhisthana chakra, Manipura chakra and again to Mooladhara chakra. Once consciousness has stabilized in the Manipura chakra for some time - vikshipta, it will steer further through the Anahata chakra and the Vishuddhi chakra to the Ajna chakra. In this state of consciousness – echagrata, the consciousness is completely focused and concentrated, sattvic. Further in the Sahasrara chakra one achieves the state of nirodha which is beyond the three gunas and then also sattva.

All functions in our body, mind and our environment are governed by the interaction between the three gunas. Even though one guna dominates, the other two are present all the time and affect our conscious state. We should learn to see which guna dominates and how the other two come into play and then learn to balance these to be able to control consciousness.

3:1
When yoga culminates – then the sight is established.
Tadā draṣṭuh svarūpe´vasthānam
Tada: then, drasuh: seeing – answer, upe: the basic nature of oneself, vasthanam: establish, develop.

The seeing develops in its true nature.

Self-awareness, kaivalya is the very goal of yoga in this context. It develops when the activity of chitta vritti ceases, when the mind is no longer affected by the interaction of the three gunas and when one ceases to identify with the material world.

The insight into our true nature comes from within. It is not possible to create or experience this insight in the state of consciousness where one still identifies with the self, the ego. It takes a purity of mind, complete mind control and freedom from desire to be able to reach this insight.

4:1

What else happens to Purusha?

Vátti sārūpyamitaratra

Vrtti: modification, pattern, sarupyam: identification, itaratra: other state.

Otherwise, there is an identification with the movements of the mind.

When the movements of the mind, chitta vrittis are not in the state of nirodha – have not calmed down, Purusha can not become aware of himself. Instead, there is an identification with chitta and its fluctuations.

When there is no awareness of the pure consciousness, Purusha, we identify with the movements of the chitta and are controlled by emotions such as feeling angry, sad or scared.

Patanjali describes different techniques that are adapted to the different needs of individuals, depending on temperament, to lead chitta to the state of nirodha. It is a prerequisite for Purusha to become aware of its true nature.

5:1

Vrittis - main divisions.

Vṛttayah pañchatayyah kliṣṭāakliṣṭāh

Vrttayah: modification of the mind, pañchatayyah: fivefold, klista: painful, difficult, aklistah: not painful.

The modification of the mind is fivefold, these are either painful or not.

There are five types of vrittis and these are either painful or non-painful. In total, there are ten types of vrittis. When you experience something as pleasant e.g. when you look at a beautiful flower it is called aklishta. When you experience something painful and uncomfortable, it is called klishta.

According to Patanjali, everything we see, hear, think and feel are different formations of the mind. According to the yogic system, all our thoughts, knowledge and various planes of consciousness are vrittis as well as our dreams.

6:1
Five types of vrittis.

Pramāṇa-viparyaya-vikalpa-nidrā smṛtayah

Pramana: right knowledge, viparyaya: wrong knowledge, vikalpa: imagination, nidra: sleep, smrtayah: memory.

The five different patterns of the mind are right knowledge, wrong knowledge, imagination, sleep and memory.

Our mind is made up of five different types of vrittis; correct knowledge, false knowledge, imagination, deep sleep and memory. These five build up the mind and shape the three dimensions of the individual consciousness. All states of mind belong to these five types of sensory patterns or vrittis (wakefulness, dreams, seeing, speaking, hearing, touching, crying, feeling and doing).

The ultimate goal of yoga is to break down these manifestations of the pattern of consciousness, ie. vrittis.

12:1

The importance of abhyasa and vairagya.

Abhyāsavairāgyābhyām tannirodhah

Abhyasa: continuous practice, vairagyabhyam: through, vairagya, tat: it, nirod-hah: stills.

Calming the five-movement patterns of the mind takes place through regular exercise and vairagya.

Patanjali describes two ways to stop the flow of chitta vrittis. Abhyasa and vairagya. Abhyasa means regular exercise. Vairagya aims at liberation from raga and dweshta ie. attraction and reluctance, to like/dislike. If you have control over these, meditation will be easier.

15:1

A lower state of vairagya.

Dṛṣṭānuśravika-viṣayāvitṛṣṇasya vaśīkāra-sañjñā vairāgyam

Drsta: the seen, anusravika: the heard, visaya: object, vitrsnasya: of the one who is free from desire, vasikara: control, sañjña: consciousness, vairagyam: absence of desire.

The state of consciousness is when the individual becomes free from the desire to satisfy the mind with what has previously been experienced and what one has heard of is vairagya.

When one is free from desire when one no longer longs for pleasure and pleasures that one has experienced in life is called vairagya. One is free from desire in the face of all objects of the mind.

It is possible to achieve vairagya even if one lives in a normal society and has family and job. It is not necessary to give up these. However, what you absolutely must give up completely is raga and dweshta.

Vairagya starts from within ourselves, not from outside. It does not matter what clothes you wear or which people you live with. What matters is what kind of attitude you have towards the events and people you meet in life. Vairagya is divided into three stages. In the first step, you are fully aware of the desires and unwillingness that you carry and you work to get over raga and dweshta. In the second stage, some objects of raga and dweshta have been taken over, but there is still something left. In the third stage, the mind is completely free from these, but they can remain latent in the subconscious.

16:1

A higher state of vairagya.

Tatparam puruṣakhyāterguṇavaitṛṣṇyam

Tat: it, param: supreme, purusakhyateh: true knowledge of purusha, gunavaitrsnyam: free from the lusts of gunas.

The highest is when one becomes free from the lusts of gunas with the knowledge of Purusha.

Once one has reached this higher state of vairagya, there is no longer a need to experience pleasure and enjoyment, acquire knowledge or be dependent on sleep. This state of vairagya is achieved when one becomes aware of Purusha.

21:1

The strength of curiosity is faster.

Tåvrasamveganāmāsannah

Tlvra: intensity, samvega: curiosity, asannah: close.

Those who carry a strong curiosity and desire, samvega, achieve asamprajnata samadhi soon.

One realizes that everything is perishable, which is a prerequisite for wanting to seek the truth.

23:1

The degree of curiosity and devotion to Ishwara (God).

Mṛdumadhyādhimātratvāt tato'pi viśeṣah

Mrdu: small, madhya: medium, adhimatra: strong, tvat: dependent on, tatopi: even, more than, viseah: specific.

As the desire grows in intensity from being small to becoming strong, asamprajnata samadhi can be achieved faster. God refers to a superior spiritual consciousness. It is neither physical nor mental but only spiritual. The highest manifested consciousness in man. According to Patanjali, if you find it difficult to develop spiritually through the techniques described, you can also do so by devoting yourself intensely to God.

28:1

Sadhana for Ishvara.

Tajjapastadarthabhāvanam

Tat: it, japa: repetition of the word, tat: it, artha: meaning, bhavanam: filled with mental.

To recite Aum and fill the mind with its meaning.

What separates Ishwara and man is that man is the manifested state of consciousness while Ishwara is the highest state of consciousness. The manifested condition continues to be manifested through rebirths, and incarnations and takes shape in various bodies such as humans and animals. When it reaches the highest stage of evolution, it takes shape in a finer and more developed body. Ishvara is beyond manifestation, of life and death and is therefore seen as the guru of the departed masters and prophets.

One cannot reach Ishwara by thinking or speaking, nor by our intellect. Thinking and experiencing are two different things. The whole Indian philosophical system is divided into tattwa chintana, a reflection of the highest consciousness, and tattwa darshan, an experience of the highest consciousness. India's six philosophical systems are based on tattwa chintana ie. knowledge. Tattwa darshan, experience, develops through yoga, bhakti, mystery and occult rituals.

Aum is like a means of expression for Ishwara, which is otherwise completely formless. This is described in yantra, mantra and tantra. These three are the expressions of the formless. Mantra is like a term in the form of sound. Pure consciousness is denoted and described in terms of the power of sound. In tantra, there is symbolism in the form of humans and animals. Yantra is a mental symbol. Aum is both a mantra and a yantra. It is not tantra as it must have a human form and have no sound.

We cannot experience Ishwara with our eyes or ears, but we experience it within ourselves using a mantra. Aum denotes Ishvara.

Through constant repetition of the word Aum – as well as dhyana about its meaning, the meditation becomes complete. Japa is not enough but must go hand in hand with meditation. Patanjali recommends that at the same time during the rehearsal of Aum one should be aware of japa and its significance. Therefore, it is important to understand the meaning of Aum. It is made up of three letters A-u-m. A relates to the world we perceive with our senses and body. U relates to the subconscious mind. M relates to the unconscious mind. By understanding this and repeating the mantra, one can change the three states of manifested consciousness, go beyond these and finally reach the fourth and mysterious stage of consciousness called turiya ie. the unmanifest state of Purusha.

30-32:1

Obstacles that may appear during sadhana and how to get past them.

1. Disease.

2. Lethargy.

3. Well-being.

4. Lack of action.

5. Laziness.

6. Strong desires.

7. Wrong perception.

8. Instability.

9. Shaking.

10. Pain.

11. Depression.

It is important to know and be prepared that difficulties and obstacles are part of the sadhana's path. When the consciousness is turned inwards, the metabolism and functions of the body change. You may fall asleep during meditation or have different perceptual experiences.

It can often seem that the person does not care about their personal life, family and other chores. You may experience doubts, and feel unsure if the sadhana is the right one or if you will reach the goal at all.

To get rid of obstacles, you need to focus on one principle – a mantra or a symbol. One should therefore stick to a certain mantra or symbol and not change it. Otherwise, the obstacles will become a fact.

There is no real difference between the different symbols, but if you change the symbol, confusion is created in the mind.

33:1

Creating Opposite Virtues - The Four Attitudes.

Maitrīkarunāmuditopeksānam sukhaduhkhapunyāpuṇyaviṣayāṇām bhāvanātaśchittaprasādanam

Maitri: kindness, karuna: compassion, mudito: joy, upeksanam: indifference, sukha: happiness, duhkha: suffering, punya: virtue, apunya: burden, visayanam: goal, bhavanatah: attitude, chitta: mind, prasadanam: pure.

To concentrate the mind, it must first be purified and stilled. This is done by developing attitudes of kindness, compassion, joy and indifference and respect for individuals as well as events that create joy, suffering, virtues or mistakes.

Through these attitudes which are:

1. Friendship with the happy.
2. Compassion for the unfortunate.
3. Gratitude and joy for what goes well.
4. Indifference to what goes wrong.

This creates a calm and undisturbed mind. It is part of the nature of the mind to be drawn to the outside world. It is not part of the nature of the mind to look inward. When turning the mind inward, one must first remove obstacles and impurities. These four attitudes remove these obstacles both on a conscious but also and unconscious level.

34:1

Control of prana.

Prachchhardanavidhāraṇābhyām vā prāṇasya

Prachchhardana: rechaka, vidharaan, bhyam: kumbakha, va: eller, pranasya; breathing.

By prolonging and keeping the spirit out, one can control the mind.

The whole mental structure consists of four different parts. Depending on the individual's temperament, different yoga paths fit differently.

1. Karma Yoga – dynamic people.

2. Bhakti yoga – emotional individuals.

3. Raya, Kriya, Swara yoga – psychic.

4. Jnana Yoga – intellectual persons.

We are often a mixture of all of these and can benefit from practicing all paths. We should choose a sadhana that suits us best to create as little resistance as possible along the way.

Patanjali describes pranayama and how by keeping the spirit inside and out of the body and through three locks we can calm our mind. He describes maha bandha where you do jalandhara, uddiyana and moola bandha while keeping your breath out. If you are a beginner, you can practice rechaka and kapalbhati, to begin with.

With the help of these exercises, the mind is calmed. It is said that the mind has two supports: prana and vasana. These are supports on which the mind rests and the consciousness works. If you delete one of these, the other also disappears automatically.

Pranan can be both rough and subtle. The subtle pran exists in the form of energy and the coarse pran is our breathing.

There are five main prana vayu that we have touched on before prana, apana, udana, samana and vyana vayu. There are also five smaller pranas: devatta, nada, kurma, krikara and dhananjaya. All of these control different parts of the body's functions:

Prana controls our inhalation and acts in the mouth and nose, digests food, separates nutrients from food, converts the water in the body into sweat and urine and controls the secretion of the glands. Its area is between the heart and the nose.

The apana removes impurities and residues from the body and has a downward movement. Its area is around the navel and feet.

Samana works in our limbs and nadis. It acts in the area around the heart and navel.

Udana maintains our muscular strength and the energy that prevails when our karmic body leaves our physical body during the moment of death. It acts in the area around the neck and head.

Vyana controls blood circulation and moves through our nerves.

Nada controls coughing and sneezing, kurma controls contractions, krikara controls hunger and thirst, devatta creates drowsiness and sleep and dhananjaya maintains nutrition.

There are also fine channels in the body called nadis. Through these, prana/impulses and signals flow to and from the brain. In total, we have about seventy-two thousand different nadis.

Ida, pingala and sushuman are the three most important of all nadis, of which sushumna is the most important channel for spiritual consciousness. These three start from the Mooladhara chakra and meet in the Ajna chakra.

Our breathing controls our thoughts in the present, past and future. During the day, breathing alternates through the right and left nostrils. You usually breathe for one hour through the right nostril and then one hour through the left nostril and about twelve times a day through each. The left nostril is called the ida and the right is the pingala. When the breathing changes from pingala to ida or from ida to pingala, the sushumna flows temporarily.

Performing heavy work is best suited when pingala nadi is flowing. When ida *nadi flows, lighter work is best suited. When sushumna nadi flows, meditation is best suited. We can control the flow through the nostrils with the help of various exercises.*

35:1

Pay attention to sensory experiences.

Viṣayavatī vā pravṛttirutpannā manasah sthitinibandhanī

Visayavati: sensual, va: or, pravrttih: functioning, panning: arises, manasah: of the mind, sthiti: steadfastness, nibandhani: which binds.

The mind can be made steady by keeping it active with sensory experiences.

If you experience that Ishwara pranidhara, maha bandha or pranayama is difficult to practice, you can instead use different sensory experiences such as sight, hearing, smell, taste and touch to create a steady and calm mind.

Nada yoga (antar mouna).
Trataka.
Kirtan.
Mantra.

36:1

Experience the inner light – optional meditation on what the mind is drawn to naturally.

Viśokā vā jyotiṣmatī

Visoka: without sorrow, va: or, jyotismati: filled with light.

The state beyond grief when filled with light can control the mind.

The mind can also be calmed by experiencing the inner peace and light between the eyebrows, bhrumadhya or by nada, concentration on sound. This inner light is calm, still and peaceful and is experienced during deep meditation.

MEDITATION

Meditation aims to establish contact with his inner self and increase his self-awareness. The goal is to realize oneself. When a person achieves self-realization, he/she has contact with his / her innermost self and identifies his or her existence – his / her life, based on his / her true self and not based on his / her ego. During meditation, one tries to establish an observed self, which means that you study your thoughts objectively and neutrally. To thus gain a perspective on oneself, one's thoughts, feelings and one's existence.

It can be said that the purpose of meditation is to explore the different regions of the mind, learn how the mind works and train it to finally surpass the mind completely. In practical terms, it can be said that meditation is about emptying the mind of thoughts, by concentrating on the present through an activity or method.

ACTIVE MEDITATION

Active meditation means that you use breathing together with some form of movement, to calm the thoughts and get into the present. Examples of active meditation are yoga, qigong and tai chi. Active meditation can also be part of our everyday life in the form of walks, eating, etc. if you do it with presence. How to put your feet up and breathe. How it feels in the body, etc.

PASSIVE MEDITATION

Passive meditation – which most people may associate with meditation, means that you sit down in silence to practice some form of meditation technique. One trains the mind through a specific method or technique to put oneself in a meditative state.

Unlike in the past, research has recently begun to look at the holistic aspect of man a little more. Research on meditation has today increased enormously unli-

ke before. The reason for this may be the increased mental disorders and diseases that are today a public health problem in many countries. The current research that has been done on yoga and meditation, shows clear and measurable results on stress-related problems such as neck and back problems, headaches, depression, anxiety, weight problems and difficulty sleeping.

To overcome these mental problems, meditation has become an increasingly recommended and used method. More and more psychologists today advise their clients to practice meditation to e.g. get in touch with their inner self and their emotions. Psychology has now come to believe that the normal stage of a human being is a constant joy.

In research on meditation, pulsating electrical voltages are measured, which the brain gives rise to so-called brain waves. These brain waves are measured via EEG (Electro Encephalo Gram: electric-brain registration). These waves can display different frequencies and these frequencies are divided into four stages. The first stage is called beta waves and are the ones we have during our normal waking state. Alpha waves are the second stage and we are then relaxed and have a state of mind that is a milder state than meditation. We have theta waves when we dream. Children, on the other hand, maybe in this stage when awake, but it is less common in adults. Delta waves are likened to deep sleep (without dreams). An experienced yogi can during meditation go from beta waves to delta waves. Research has also shown that those who have practiced meditation for a long time have more stable brain waves (have constant coherence) and a greater mental balance, which i.a. triggers endorphins that strengthen the immune system.

Physiologically, meditation reduces muscle tension, improves respiratory rhythm, digestion, immune system, blood pressure and heart rate and increases the efficiency of the internal organs.

Many people who meditate regularly experience that they get more energy, be-

come more alert, and sleep better, the stress level in the body decreases, concentration and the ability to focus are strengthened and the ability to perform and oxygen uptake is improved.

The autonomic nervous system is divided into the sympathetic nervous system and the parasympathetic nervous system. The sympathetic nervous system is usually called the "fight or flight defense system", which is the system that is activated during mental or physical stress. When this is activated, the pupils dilate, blood pressure increases, digestion decreases, and blood sugar increases. The parasympathetic nervous system is the opposite, it is activated when the body is at rest. It lowers blood pressure, stimulates digestion, improves the body's healing processes and it secretes oxytocin (the body's own calm and growth hormone). These two systems complement each other.

Today's society and the life we live today result in the sympathetic nervous system being activated in many people almost all the time. The sympathetic nervous system is meant to be activated only for short periods, but as today's threats often consist of fears of not being able to pay bills, worries about the job, etc., it leads to it often being activated for a longer period. This leads to people always being tense, unhappy and having a harder time resisting illness. If the sympathetic nervous system is activated, it can also lead to high blood pressure, diabetes, heart attack and several mental disorders linked to stress.

The only way to prevent this is through relaxation, both physically and mentally and of course with good sleep. Meditation provides both physical and mental relaxation. We must also learn to react differently to our surroundings and what we are exposed to in our everyday lives so that the adrenaline content does not increase at all possible times.

THINKING ABOUT MEDITATION

When sitting down for meditation, it is important to think about a few things. The first preparation is that you can sit undisturbed, in a place where you feel silence. Turn off all phones and make sure no one is disturbed. The morning or before bedtime are the best times for meditation. Also remember not to eat too close to the meditation, as the body is full of digestion and a lot of blood and energy is drawn in from the body to the stomach.

Then make sure you have something to sit on, a meditation pillow, a regular pillow or a chair. Take the time to find a comfortable sitting position. You must sit comfortably as you will sit still for a while. A popular sitting position is siddhasana where you sit on the buttocks with the legs outstretched, insert one foot towards the groin and the other foot you place just in front of the shin or on top of the shin. Make sure you are sitting in a three-point position where both buttocks are in contact with the ground and both knees.

You place your hands either on your knees with the palm facing down and let your thumb and forefinger meet in jnana mudra. Alternatively, place the right back of the hand in the left palm and let the thumbs meet in bhairavi mudra. It is important that you feel your hands resting securely so that you can relax your shoulders.

Feel that you are sitting with a straight spine where the weight from the upper body can fall straight down through the pelvis. Insert your chin slightly next to your chest so that your neck can relax and close your eyes. Have a little weight forward on the pelvis so that you do not collapse with your back.

Then start by landing in yourself with your thoughts and with your presence, calm the mind and relax the body with for example kaya stahairyam. Then start your chosen meditation technique with, for example, ajapa japa. It is important not to have any expectations of the meditation and what one is believed to experience.

There are also various obstacles that one may encounter during meditation, such as thoughts and feelings. There can be obstacles such as anger, pride and *selfishness, which can be trained away, among other things. Practice yamas and niyamas. If any thoughts or feelings arise during the meditation, become aware of them, see them but then let them float on with the next exhalation and then return to focusing on the chosen meditation technique.*

If you feel that it is difficult to calm down, it can be an advantage to have done something active before setting out for meditation, such as taking a walk or doing a yoga session.

It is important to have regularity in your meditation practice.

CLASSICAL TECHNIQUES FOR MEDITATION

The classic sitting positions for meditation (meditation asanas) are padmasana, siddhasana, siddha yoni asana and swastikasana. For beginners (and Westerners who are often stiff and have narrower hips) you can also sit in sukhasana or ardha padmasana. If for various reasons you need to sit on a chair, you can also do so. The principle is that the sitting position should be comfortable and provide support for the body during meditation so you can relax. It's not about sitting nicely. The back must be straight so that the prana can flow upwards in the body. You can also lie comfortably on your back, but then there is the risk of falling asleep.

Important mudras during meditation include jnana/chin mudra, bhairavi mudra and khechari mudra.

JNANA MUDRA

Place your hands on your knees with your palms facing down and let your thumb and forefinger meet.

CHIN MUDRA

Place your hands on your knees with the palm facing up and let your thumb and forefinger meet.

BHAIRAVI MUDRA

You place the right back of the hand in the left palm and let your thumbs meet.

KHECHARI MUDRA

Roll up the tongue so that you place the back of the tongue up in the palate with gentle pressure.

UJJAYI PRANAYAMA

Ujjayi pranayama also called the psychic/winning breath. Start by placing the back of the tongue up in the palate in the khechari mudra, narrow in the air passage and strive for a whispering/hissing – ah sound. Breathe through your nose but feel that the breathing and the sound come far in from the throat. It sounds a bit like when you blow mist on a mirror with an open mouth. Children usually say that the sound is similar to Darth Vader's breathing in Star Wars.

Ujjayi pranayama is used in many different meditation techniques (and also during the practice of asanas) as it has a calming effect on the nervous system and also lowers blood pressure. It also emits a sound as a focal point to draw attention to. Breathing in this way also means that you retain the heat.

BHRUMADHYA

Bhrumadhya is a point in the ajna chakra (third eye). The word itself – bhrumadhya, means eyebrow center and this is also where this point is located.

CHIDAKASHA

Chidakasha can be explained as our inner mental television screen. It is visualized as space in front of our closed eyes and this is where our psychic event/event appears – "what the mind carries". Chidakasha stands for "area of knowledge" and Akasha means space.

JAPA YOGA

Japa yoga is an effective technique for bringing the mind back to the present using the mantra. Japa means repetition of a mantra. The mantra affects us both physically and mentally, both with the help of the meaning of the word and its vibrations it states within one. Mantra meditation cleanses the subconscious mind and causes the thought activity to decrease, as the mind does not receive any new stimulus. This makes it easier to get in touch with your inner self. A constant repetition of the mantra makes the mind concentrated and relaxed and gives us inner peace. It is important not to force focus on the mantra but to let it come naturally from within. One can practice japa with different forms of mantras, it can be mantras that one pronounces aloud (baikhari), mantras to whisper (upanshu), mental mantras (mansaik), or written mantras (likhit). You often recite the mantra a certain number of times and to help you with the count you can have a mala, which is a rosary with pearls. You can practice Japa yoga both sitting in a meditation position and while performing other daily activities.

AJAPA JAPA

Ajapa japa is a complete sadhana (spiritual practice where one eventually achieves self-realization) in itself. By regularly practicing ajapa japa for a long time, subconscious desires, and fears will finally come to the surface which one will then view with a witness attitude and thus get to the root of physical and mental problems and can change them.

Japa means repetition of a mantra. Ajapa japa means constant awareness. Traditionally, the mantra So-Ham is used, but it is possible to use any mantra if, for example, you have received a mantra from your guru.

HARI OM TAT SAT

A guided meditation often ends with Hari Om Tat Sat in classical yoga.

Hari Om Tat Sat are two different mantras that have been brought together, Hari Om is one and Tat Sat is the other. Hari stands for the manifested universe and life, the energy – Shakti. Om stands for the absolute reality, the consciousness – Shiva. Reality consists of both the complete (incomprehensible) and the

126

YOGASCHITTA VRITTI NIRODHAH

(WHEN THE MOVEMENTS OF THE MIND ARE STILL, YOGA OCCURS)

LESSON NO. 3

LONG SHAVASANA – DEAD MAN'S POSTURE /RELAXATION.

PRANAYAMA – YOGIC BREATHING.

SUPTA PAWANMUKTASANA – LEG LOCK.

SURYA NAMASKARA – SUN GREETING WITHOUT BREATHING.

VAYU NISHKASANA – THE PUMP.

SHAVASANA – DEAD MAN'S POSTURE.

SHAVA UDARAKARSHANASANA – THE UNIVERSAL POSITION.

SHAVASANA – DEAD MAN'S POSTURE.

SARPASANA – THE SNAKE.

SHASHANKASANA – THE HARE.

SHAVASANA – DEAD MAN'S POSTURE.

VAJROLI, SAHAROLI & ASHWINI – MUDRAS.

YOGA NIDRA – DEEP RELAXATION.

KAYA STHAIRYAM & AJAPA JAPA – STEP 1 – MEDITATION.

END WITH – HARI OM TAT SAT, 3 TIMES.

THEN – OM SRI DURGAYAI NAMAH, 1 TIME.

INSTRUCTIONS FOR ASANAS LESSON NO 3.

LONG SHAVASANA – DEAD MAN'S POSTURE/RELAXATION.

Execution: See module 1.

PRANAYAMA – YOGIC BREATHING.

Execution: See modules 1 and 2.

SUPTA PAWANMUKTASANA – LEG LOCK.

Execution: See modules 1 and 2.

SURYA NAMASKARA – SUN SALUTATION WITHOUT BREATHING

Execution: Stand straight at the front of the mat with your feet shoulder-width apart. Place your hands in namaskar (greeting) on your chest. Stretch your arms straight up to the ceiling and lean back and salute the sun. Then bend your knees and come down to the floor with both hands. Take a big step back with your right foot. As you lower your right knee to the floor, push up high onto your fingertips and look up at the sun. Then take a big step back with your left foot and come up with the posterior towards the roof in the mountain position. Step back with both feet slightly and get down into the mask - feet, chest and chin on the floor. Tighten your buttocks. Hands next to the chest, palms downward, elbows pointing upwards towards the ceiling. Then push off with your toes and pull yourself forward a little with your hands while you move into the half cobra pose. Lift your head up high keeping your arms bent, shoulders lowered, and legs straight and close together. Keep your abdomen touching the mat. Then come up into the mountain again, step forward with your left foot and look up at the sun. Bring your back foot forward to meet your left foot, so both legs are straight and your hands are touching your feet. Then bend your knees and rise and greet the sun again and lean far back. Finish the sun salutation with your hands on your chest. This is a half-round. Do the same again, but this time start by moving the left foot back and then the right to the front. Practice three to six full rounds.

VAYU NISHKASANA – THE PUMP.

Execution: Squat on the floor with your feet wide apart. Slide your palms under your instep with your elbows inside your knees. Inhale and look up while pushing out your knees with your elbows, hold your breath for a while and then push your rear end up towards the ceiling and straighten your legs. Keep your hands under your feet throughout the exercise. When you stretch your legs straight and have your head down at your knees, exhale. Continue like this for a few minutes.

SHAVASANA – DEAD MAN´S POSTURE.

Execution: See module no. 1 & 2.

SHAVA UDARAKARSHANASANA – THE UNIVERSAL POSITION.

Execution: See modules 1 & 2.

SARPASANA – THE SNAKE.

Execution: See module 1.

SHASHANKASANA – THE HARE.

Execution: See modules 1 & 2.

VAJROLI, SAHAROLI & ASHWINI – MUDRAS.

Execution: Sit in any meditation position. Inhale and contract only the rectum on one inhalation. Then release the ashwini mudra with an exhale. Continue for about 3-5 minutes or longer. Then continue with vajroli (men) & saharoli (women) mudra. Same technique, but now pinch the genitals together on inhalation instead. Same length.

YOGA NIDRA *(nidra: sleep)*

YOU INTRODUCE

Get ready for yoga nidra.

Lie down in the shavasana and straighten your clothes, so you lie comfortably and do feel the need to move again.

Now, concentrate on the body.

Become aware of the silence of the body.

You lie completely still as if your body were made of stone.

Aware of the body – body awareness.

Listen to all the sounds around you.

All sounds simultaneously, effortlessly.

Tell yourself ... I'm awake and going to practice yoga nidra, I'm not going to fall asleep.

Now it's time to make your Sankalpa. Your inner wish. Your decision for this yoga nidra.

Positive, clear and distinct – 3 times, you say it quietly to yourself.

It goes deep into your subconscious and is bound to manifest.

Repeat the body parts after me in your head and fill them with your consciousness – go to your right hand ...

Thumb on your right side, index finger, middle finger, ring finger, little finger, hand, arm, shoulder, armpit, chest, abdomen, thigh, knee, shin, foot, big toe, second toe, third toe, fourth toe and so little toe, feel the whole of your right side ...

Take your consciousness to your left side ... feel your left thumb, index finger etc...

Feel the back of your head, neck, shoulders, spine, entire back ... buttocks, thighs, back knees, calves, feet ... Feel the entire back of your body ...

Feel the top of the head, forehead, nose, tip of the nose, lips, chin tip, neck, collarbone, chest, arms, navel, inside the navel, genitals, thighs, knees, shins, feet, toes ...

Feel the whole right arm, the whole left arm, the whole right leg, left leg, torso, head ... the whole body ...

Concentrate now on breathing ... experience it, do not control it ... go to the left nostril, feel how you draw in air and how it goes out through the right nostril ... feel the temperature difference at the upper lip ...

On 1 you draw in air through the left nostril, on 1 out through the right, on 2 in through the right and 2 out through the left ... on 5, 10, 15 etc. you draw in air through both nostrils and out through both. Count carefully, if you count incorrectly, start again from 1 ... (anuloma, viloma & prana shuddhi - alternating breathing) ...

See the following objects in front of you, touch them, smell them ... a desert, pyramid, temple, a Buddha statue, a rose, waves far out to sea, candle flame, sunrise, birds flying, clouds ... yin and yang, Shiva, a triangle with the tip down, a triangle with the tip up, lying on top of each other so they form a six-pointed star, a circle, a square, experience happiness, a golden egg, a pulsating white glow at the center of the eyebrows ... a daisy lotus flower on top of your head ...

Now it's time to repeat your decision, your sankalpa - clearly, 3 times ...

I say Hari Om Tat Sat 3 times and then yoga nidra is over for this time

TERMINATION

Hari Om Tat Sat 3 times.

... we can now open our eyes and start moving our bodies ...

TIME & ADVICE

Yoga nidra can be anywhere from 15-45 minutes long. You can build on this with chakra visualizations, experiences of yantra and deepen the exercise depen-

ding on the purpose and experience of the group. Adjust the number of visua-
lizations to the time you have available, but always go through the body parts
as usual without stress. Make sure that the participants do not lie on yoga mats
that are too hard or thin or get cold. It can be an advantage to use a blanket and
something soft under the back of the head. Ask participants to stretch a forearm
in the air if they tend to fall asleep. If the arm falls, they wake up.

KAYA STHAIRYAM

Show alternative meditation postures in the first lesson. One can practice kaya
sthairyam without ajapa japa. Then use a similar finish as in ajapa japa.

HOW TO INTRODUCE

Sit in a comfortable meditation position and pay attention to your body. Spend
some time adjusting your position, check your legs and feet are positioned
correctly, and change your position now if you need to, before meditation begins.
Choose the position with care, you should be able to sit in it as comfortably as
possible for the next 20 minutes ...

Take a deep breath and at the same time stretch the whole spine up to the ceiling.
When exhaling, relax, but keep the stretch in the back. Relax the facial muscles,
forehead, eyelids, cheeks, lips, tongue, and lower jaw. Relax your arms, and let
your hands rest on your knees or inside your knees completely relaxed. Relax
your buttocks, legs and feet ...

Feel the contact between the surface you are sitting on and the parts of your
body that rest on it. Be aware of your body position and try to visualize it. Your
body is alive, a lot is happening in it right now, pay attention to the different
emotions that your body signals ...

Now take all your attention to the right leg, creating an inner image of the whole
leg in the position it is in. Be aware of how it feels in the leg, from the toes up
to the buttocks. Is there any pressure, pain, stretching, heat, cold, or any other
feeling? Focus your attention on this for a while ...

Now shift your attention to the left leg, try to visualize it, and again, feel how it
feels throughout the leg. What can you feel right now? If you notice tension, relax

in that part. Continue in the same way with the abdomen, chest, whole back, arms, head (especially the face) ...

Now visualize your whole body, try to see a clear picture of your body in a meditation position, steady and immobile as a statue ...

Now also be aware of breathing. Your body is breathing and you are witnessing it. Natural relaxed breathing, which you observe with the utmost care. You know you are inhaling, you know you are exhaling ...

Be aware of the movement of the stomach ... be aware of the movement of the chest ... be aware of the passage of air through the nostrils ...

Finish by making a smooth transition to ajapa japa.

AJAPA JAPA

STEP 1. RESPIRATORY CONSCIOUSNESS

Move your awareness between different parts and aspects of breathing.

YOU INTRODUCE

You experience the movement in the abdomen and the chest ... the stomach expanding on inhalation ... the stomach contracting on exhalation ...

You experience airflow through both nostrils ... calm even rhythm ...

You are aware of the sound of breathing ... natural rhythm.

STEP 2. ACTIVATE THE YOGIC BREATH

An exercise focusing on the movement of the breath in a passage between the navel and the neck ...

Hold the breath at the neck ... say vishuddhi 3 times, then breathe down to the navel ... hold the breath out ... say manipura 3 times ... then breathe up to the neck ... etc.

STEP 3. UJJAYI PRANAYAMA

Activate ujjayi pranayama and khechari mudra.

STEP 4. MANTRA SO-HAM

Be fully aware of the mantra in coordination with breathing ...
SO...O with inhalation ... HA ... AM with exhalation.

AWARENESS OF THOUGHTS

If thoughts or feelings arise spontaneously: be aware of them, but then let them
disappear as if on small clouds...

Remind yourself of this several times during ongoing meditation. Try your best
to develop an active and conscious attitude.

TERMINATION

Hari Om Tat Sat 3 times.

We can return to our natural breathing, stop the experience of the passage and
our two chakras, stop the mantra and gently open our eyes and start moving the
body...

SWADHISTHANA CHAKRA (YOU CAN READ ABOUT THE CHAKRA-NA IN MODUL 4)

To practice regularly for a month.

Chakra and kshetram localization, activation and purification. For the chakra:
Ashwini mudra – first slowly. Inhale, contract the rectum and hold the breath...
feel the pulsation with Vam in the chakra a few centimeters up from the end of
the tailbone... then quickly and with Vam in time with breathing.

For kshetram: Vajroli (or sahajoli) mudra – first slowly. Inhale and contract the
genitals and hold your breath... feel the pulsation with Vam at the kshetram for
the chakra at the genitals ... then quickly and with Vam in time with breathing.

KNOWLEDGE TEST MODULE 3

ANSWER AS FULLY AS YOU CAN, THEN CHECK IF YOU ANSWERED CORRECTLY. PRACTICE UNTIL YOU KNOW THE ANSWERS BY HEART.

1. DESCRIBE THE THREE GUNAS.

2. DESCRIBE WHAT AUM IS.

3. EXPLAIN THE BASICS OF VIVEKA AND YOGA PHILOSOPHY.

4. WHAT ARE THE YOGA SUTRAS?

5. DESCRIBE WHAT MEDITATION IS.

6. WHAT SHOULD ONE THINK ABOUT IN MEDITATION?

7. DESCRIBE THE CLASSICAL TECHNIQUES FOR MEDITATION.

8. WHAT ARE CLASSIC YOGA AND RAJA YOGA?

9. DESCRIBE THE SWADHISTHANA CHAKRA, ITS ELEMENT, YANTRA, COLOR, NUMBER OF PETALS AND ATTRIBUTES.

10. DESCRIBE SOME POWERFUL EXERCISES TO ACTIVATE, CLEAN AND BALANCE SWADHISTHANA CHAKRA.

MODULE 4

KUNDALINI YOGA. WE STUDY KUNDALINI SHAKTI AND THE CHAKRA SYSTEM AND LEARN THE PRINCIPLES BEHIND AWAKING OUR LATENT POWERS

We study Kundalini Shakti and her various names and immerse ourselves in the chakra system and its inherent forces and influence on our life potential. We are also beginning to approach Kriya yoga. We study the Manipura chakra and practice our own exercises to cleanse, balance and activate the chakra. We continue to practice in the role of yoga teacher with lesson no. 4 of 8.

Knowledge test: Answer the questions related to module 4. Practice lesson no. 4 with at least 1 participant and humbly accept feedback from them. Ask questions afterward – how was the pace, did you keep to time, did you speak loudly enough, and how well did you understand the exercises?

KUNDALINI YOGA

WHAT IS KUNDALINI?

Kundalini is what we call the dormant energy that exists in every human being. It has its seat at the bottom of the spine in the perineum or pelvic floor, (between the urine and the excretory organs) in men and at the cervix (the bottom of the cervix in women). This is also where the Mooladhara chakra is found.

With the help of yogic techniques such as asana, pranayama, Kriya yoga and meditation, one can increase the flow of prana in the body and direct it down to Mooladhara to awaken the Kundalini Shakti. When the Kundalini energy then begins to rise upwards along the Sushumna nadi and through the chakras, the dormant parts of the brain that are in contact with the respective chakras are awakened. Through this process, we can have greater access to the capacity of our brain and raise our consciousness.

The awakening of Kundalini should be done slowly and systematically. The body and mind should be prepared slowly. This way, you avoid any risks that a rise may entail. One should not try to control or influence the mind as such. The mind is an "extension" of the body and therefore it is easiest to start with the body and gradually move on with prana, nadis and chakras.

HOW THE KUNDALINI WAS DISCOVERED

Since the beginning, man has been involved in, and experienced events of a supernatural nature. When it so happened that one would feel what others were thinking and wanting, the inner visions manifested and dreams came true. It was noticed that a certain crowd of people had a very special ability to express their creativity through art, music and poetry. Some people had a strong drive, and zest for life while others barely managed to get up in the morning. Man became curious as to what was the cause of these differences. In the end, through one's own experience, one could conclude that in man there was a special form of energy. In some, this energy was dormant, in development in others, and fully awakened in very few. This energy was called after gods and deities. After they also discovered prana, they started calling it prana Shakti. In Tantrism, this energy is called Kundalini Shakti.

DIFFERENT NAMES

In Sanskrit, Kundalini means "spiral" or "something that is rolled up". Kundalini Shakti has thus traditionally been described as something that has just been rolled up. Nevertheless, the meaning of the whole thing has often been misunderstood. Kundalini derives from the word – kunda, which refers to "a deeper place", or a pit. The place where a dead body is burned is also called a customer. The word Kundalini refers to Shakti, or the power, energy in its dormant state. When it then wakes up and manifests itself, it is called Devi, Kali, Durga, Saraswati, Lakshmi or something else depending on the characteristics and qualities that it evokes in man.

In Christianity, terms such as "the path of the initiated" or "the stairs to heaven" are used. These refer to the Kundalini that rises along the sushumna. The Christian cross symbolizes Kundalini rising and the resulting spiritual beauty. In all spiritual paths, whether one is talking about samadhi, nirvana, moksha, unity, kaivalya or liberation, it is the Kundalini awakening one is referring to.

KUNDALINI, DURGA, KALI

When you can positively handle a raised Kundalini, its quality is called Durga. If Kundalini instead wakes up when you are still unprepared and not ready to handle it, it is called Kali.

The goddess Kali is illustrated as naked, black and she wears a rosary of one hundred and eight human skulls that represent memories from previous lives. Her blood-red outstretched tongue symbolizes rajo guna whose circular movement pattern gives power to all creative activity. She wants to urge sadhakas to take control of rajo guna.

Durga is a beautiful goddess who is illustrated riding a tiger. She has eight arms that represent the eightfold elements. She wears a rosary with fifty-two human skulls that symbolize her wisdom, power and the fifty-two letters of the Sanskrit alphabet. Durga eliminates all the evil consequences that life can carry with it and comes with power and peace. This force is released from Mooladhara.

KUNDALINI PHYSIOLOGY

When Kundalini begins to rise, it passes different phases on its way up to the cosmic consciousness – Shiva, where they finally merge. The highest consciousness – Shiva, has its seat in Sahasrara - the super consciousness, at the top of the head. In the Vedic texts as well as in Tantrism, this seat is called Hiranyagarbha – the womb of consciousness. It is connected to the pituitary gland. Just below there is another psychic center called the Ajna chakra which is connected to the pineal gland, the seat of intuitive consciousness. It is located at the top of the spine and the height of the eyebrow center – bhrumadhya. Ajna chakra is important as it is connected to both Mooladhara and Sahasrara chakra.

Chakras are energy vortices that are experienced to vibrate and rotate at different speeds. There are thousands of chakras in the human body. In tantra and yoga, only a few are used for filling the entire spectrum of human evolution and life – physically and mentally, from the rough to the polished. Six chakras have a direct connection to the dormant parts of the brain.

Through nadis, energy flows to and from the chakras. Nadis are channels where prana (vital) and mana (mental) energy flows through and out to all parts of the body. There are about seventy-two thousand nadis. Three of these are extra important as they control the flow of prana and the consciousness of all other nadis. These are ida, pingala and sushumna. Ida controls all the mental activity and pingala all the vital activity. Ida is known as the moon and pingala as the sun. Sushumna is the channel for the flow of spiritual consciousness. Ida and pingala do not flow in the body at the same time but they alternate. When the left nostril is open, ida nadi flows and when the right nostril is open, the pingala flows. When the pingala flows, the left part of the brain is active and when the ida flows, the right part of the brain is active. In this way, nadis control our brain, way of acting and consciousness.

If you can get prana and chitta, ie. ida and pingala flow at the same time, you can also get both halves of the brain to cooperate in thinking and action. This does not happen in our normal daily lives. For this to happen, it is required that the sushumna is in contact with Kundalini Shakti.

Sushumna nadi is like a hollow tube with three more tubes in it. One is more subtle than the other. These tubes, or nadis, are called sushumna (denotes tamas), vajrini (denotes rajas), chitrini (denotes sattva) and Brahma (denotes consciousness). The highest consciousness born of Kundalini Shakti passes through Brahma.

When Kundalini wakes up, the sushumna passes up to the Ajna chakra. Mooladhara acts as a powerful engine. To start this engine, pranic energy is needed and it is created with the help of pranayamas. The prana is then directed downwards in the body, to the Mooladhara chakra. From there it is then directed upwards towards the Ajna chakra. If the sushumna nadi is not open, the energy cannot be distributed, which means that the prana remains in the Mooladhara chakra.

Ida and pingala nadi are constantly flowing but their power is weak. It is only when the sushumna is awakened that enlightenment can take place. Kundalini yoga is based on awakening the sushumna, and when awakened, contact between the highest and lowest levels of consciousness is enabled. Then Kundalini can wake up and rise from Mooladhara up along the sushumna and then become one with Shiva in Sahasrara.

THE MYSTICAL TREE

In Bhagavad Gita, you can read about the immortal tree that grows up and down, with the roots up and the leaves and branches down. It is said that he who knows the tree also knows the truth of life. This tree is found in the human body and nervous system. Thoughts, feelings, obstacles, etc. symbolized by the leaves of the tree. The brain is symbolized by the roots and the spine of the trunk. You have to climb from the top of the tree (in this case from the root) and up to the roots. In Kabbalah, this tree is called the "tree of life". In the Bible it is called the "tree of knowledge." Anyone who tries to move upwards from Mooladhara to Sahasrara thus climbs to the roots.

KUNDALINI AND OUR BRAIN

Humans are often said to use only a tenth of the full capacity of the brain. The knowledge we have, what we think and do is stored in this small part. The rest is known as the dormant and inactive part of the brain. The reason it is inactive is that the amount of energy is not enough to keep it awake. The active part of the brain gets its energy from ida and pingala nadi while the dormant part only has access to pingala ie. prana, or, life energy. It lacks conscious energy, ie. ida, or, manas.

To awaken the sleeping part of the brain, we must charge the front part of the brain with prana and consciousness. We must also awaken sushumna nadi. We do this by practicing pranayamas regularly for an extended period. With the help of Kundalini yoga, one could discover that the different parts of the brain were connected to our chakras. To access dormant parts of the brain, one must work on awakening the chakras in the body. Chakras can be described as switches.

In the same way, the Mooladhara chakra is used as a "switch" to awaken Kundalini, which has its seat in Sahasrara, but most of us find it easier to get in touch with Mooladhara. Each chakra works individually. This means that if Kundalini wakes up in Mooladhara, it goes straight from there up to Sahasrara. Or, if it wakes up in Swadhisthana, it also goes from there straight up to Sahasrara. Kundalini can be awakened in a chakra or collectively in all chakras at the same time. When Kundalini awakens in an individual chakra, the consciousness is filled with what is characteristic of that particular chakra.

WHAT KUNDALINI SHAKTI IS

There are many different descriptions of what Kundalini Shakti is. Many yogis believe that Kundalini Shakti is pranic energy that flows through the sushumna associated with the spine. They believe that Kundalini is part of the pranic flow in our energy body and that there is no physical/anatomical equivalent.

Other yogis experience Kundalini as part of the signals that flow along the nerve pathways and that travel along the spinal cord up to specific parts of the brain. However, most agree that the experience of Kundalini is something psychophysiological that is manifested in the spine.

METHODS FOR AWAKENING:

In Tantrism, various techniques are used to awaken Kundalini Shakti. These can be practiced individually or in combination with each other.

AWAKENED IN CONNECTION WITH BIRTH

A few children are born with an already awake Kundalini. These children look at life very clearly, and have a highly developed way of thinking and a very unusual way of looking at life. They often have no normal social relationship with their parents because they see them as "those who gave them life".

MANTRA

It is a powerful, gentle and risk-free method. However, it requires patience, time, discipline and regularity. Through mantra repetition and the vibration of sound, a wave of patterns is created that affects the mind. The physical, mental and emotional body is cleansed. It is important to focus the mantra on something by, for example, focusing on the tip of the nose or a chakra.

TAPASYA

It is a psychological procedure where you start a process that from the root eliminates bad habits that have created weakness and hinder development and willpower. Willpower is the core of tapasya. To enable the development and willpower, you want to curb the inner fire, live in celibacy, say no to lust, be restrained and, deny your desires.

ASUHADHI – *Using Herbs*

This is the fastest and most effective method besides tantric initiation. It should not be confused with the use of drugs. Asuhadhi is a risky method that should only be done under the guidance of a guru.

RAJA YOGA

With Raja yoga, one merges the individual consciousness with the universal superconscious. This is done step by step with the help of concentration, meditation and the experience of unity with the absolute and highest self. When you focus and calm your mind, the sushumna opens, which enables the rising of Kundalini. This is a mild method that is experienced to be difficult by many because it requires a lot of patience and discipline.

PRANAYAMA

Pranayamas are very powerful. If you are well prepared, live healthy, and have a calm and safe place to practice breathing exercises, Kundalini can be awakened very quickly. Pranayamas strongly affect the body, creating heat while lowering the temperature in the inner body. Breathing changes the pattern of brain waves. It is important to cleanse the body with the help of shatkarmas before entering the process to better handle the rapid changes that come. Breathing is the link between Hatha and Kundalini yoga.

KRIYA YOGA

This is the simplest method for people living in the modern world. Here you do not have to confront the mind as in e.g. Raja yoga. People who are Sattvic may find it easy to awaken Kundalini through Raja yoga, but if you have a tumultuous mind that is constantly in motion, it only creates even more tension, guilt, complex and sometimes even schizophrenia. When practicing Kriya yoga, Kundalini Shakti is awakened slowly and methodically.

TANTRIC INITIATION

This method requires an understanding of what Shiva and Shakti stand for. You have to change your approach to passions and desires in life. Under the guidance of a guru, this is the fastest way to Kundalini awakening.

SHAKTIPAT

This method is performed by a guru. One experiences a temporary state of awakening – samadhi.

SURRENDER YOURSELF

This path means that one does not strive to awaken Kundalini Shakti. You let it happen when it happens and if it happens. It is believed that a strong enough will can arouse Kundalini.

PREPARATIONS

It is important to learn Kundalini yoga from a competent teacher so that one knows for sure that the process is going the right way. It is also important to be physically, mentally and emotionally prepared. Waking up Kundalini Shakti can take time and you can count on it being a long process. However, there is nothing that says that Kundalini cannot wake up quickly. What takes time is learning to keep the Kundalini alive.

The sushumna must be open, otherwise, Kundalini will rise along the ida or pingala which leads to complications. The elements, chakras and nadis must also be purified for Kundalini to flow freely. This is done with the help of asanas, pranayamas and Hatha yoga shatkarmas.

Surya namaskar and surya bheda pranayama cleanses pingala nadi. Shatkarmas and pranayamas open up the sushumna. You start by cleaning the elements with shatkarma. Then continue with asanas and pranayamas. After that, you can continue with mudras and bandhas. Then you are ready to start with Kriya yoga.

KARMA YOGA

Karma yoga is a very important part of spiritual development. Without Karma yoga, evolution will stop no matter what method one chooses to follow. Karma yoga prepares the mind. Positive and negative partners become visible, consciousness is broadened and concentration is strengthened. Karma yoga is not a direct cause of Kundalini awakening but an important part of the process.

DIFFERENT AWAKENINGS

It is important to be able to distinguish between the awakening of Kundalini, chakras and sushumna nadi. It should also be possible to distinguish between an awakening between Mooladhara and Kundalini. The first step in awakening Kundalini Shakti is to create harmony between ida and pingala nadi. The next step is to awaken the chakra system which leads to the sushumna opening and which allows for the Kundalini Shakti to wake up.

When the process takes place in this order, you do not have to worry about negative consequences. If Kundalini instead wakes up before the sushumna is open, the energy will remain in the Mooladhara chakra and create sexual and neurotic disorders. Should any chakra not be open, Kundalini will get stuck in its path and create stagnation in development.

Harmony between ida and pingala nadi:

Pingala stands for vital energy in the body. Ida stands for conscious energy. These two nadis control the two hemispheres of the brain, which in turn control all activity in the body. It is not the awakening of these two that one strives for but the synchronization between them. As is well known, these control the body's temperature, digestion, hormonal secretion, brain waves and the whole body's system. Bad food and lifestyle disturbs and creates an imbalance between them, which leads to physical and mental illness. Sushumna can only wake up when ida and pingala flow in harmony. Hatha yoga, pranayamas and Raja yoga are the best methods to create harmony between ida and pingala. Especially nadi shodhana.

Awaken the chakras:

All chakras must be balanced before the sushumna can wake up. Every little part of the body is connected to a chakra. Asanas open up the chakras in a gentle way. Sometimes a chakra can open quickly. Then feelings of fear, anxiety, passion, depression, etc. can emerge that have connections to previous experiences from previous lives.

Awaken the Sushumna:

It takes a lot of patience to awaken the sushumna nadi. You can expect to have experiences of a more intense nature than those that come when a chakra is awakened. These experiences are often completely illogical and strange. Hatha yoga and pranayamas are essential for awakening sushumna nadi.

KUNDALINI SINKS IN

After a rise, Kundalini will fall again. But the mind and consciousness will still be affected and changed. You get a higher state of consciousness. Our whole lives and our thoughts are affected. Emotions, body, and mind. Kundalini will be what characterizes life.

When Shiva and Shakti become one in Sahasrara, one experiences samadhi and silent parts of the brain wake up. In this state, one is completely unaware of opposites, man and woman, Shiva and Shakti – everything is the same. During the experience of samadhi, Bindu develops. Bindu means point and encompasses the entire cosmos. It is the seat of human intelligence and all creation. After a while, the Bindu is divided into two and the duality of Shiva and Shakti becomes reality again.

Samadhi can be likened to the condition of an infant. One does not know the difference between man and woman and there is no physical or sexual difference. When Shiva and Shakti return to the rough plane, down to the Mooladhara chakra, they separate. Duality exists in the mind in the world that consists of name and form but not in samadhi.

When Kundalini sinks and you return to physical reality, you do it with a changed consciousness. You may live your life just as before, with the same patterns, desires and passions. What makes the difference is that you observe life as if it were a spectacle.

You are in the theater of life just as before but as a spectator. The changed consciousness is manifested through one. You are in contact with the parts of the brain that were previously silent. One is in contact with the knowledge, power and wisdom of the universe.

THE EXPERIENCE OF THE AWAKENING

A Kundalini rise can be likened to an explosion that takes you from one plane of consciousness to another plane of being. You travel through the borderland where perceptions, feelings and experiences change character. It is a journey between what you have experienced and the inexperienced.

The awakening takes place step by step and can take time. The preliminary awakening, and usually the first step, is the experience of light at bhrumadhya. This usually develops over a long period, in a very mild way and rarely creates any negative experiences. After a while, your appetite and need for sleep may decrease and your mind is still.

When the Kundalini rise finally takes place, it happens with power and sometimes you can experience things that are difficult to comprehend. One of the most common experiences is the feeling of "a current" along the spine. One can experience a burning sensation in Mooladhara and an energy flowing up and down along the sushumna. You can also hear sounds in the form of drums, bells, music, birds and flutes. You can also experience anger, passion and other repressed emotions that emerge. This usually passes within a few days. Some develop siddhis which after a while also disappear.

You can lose your appetite for weeks, become depressed, lose interest in life and experience everything as very sad at the same time as the mind can become very mobile and creative. You might start writing poetry, creating music or some other art. This flattens out after a while and you land in your normal life and normal life again. From the outside, everything looks like before, but you have an increased inner awareness and ability to observe. Headaches and insomnia can occur in some people when Kundalini wakes up.

It is easy to confuse the awakening of our chakras, nadis and sushumna with a Kundalini rise. When the chakra is opened, you get experiences that are usually pleasant and satisfying. They are rarely nasty or scary. When you get pleasant experiences during meditation or the kirtan or can feel the presence of your guru, it is a chakra awakening that takes place and not Kundalini.

When sushumna wakes up, you can experience the spine as shining or as a streak of light. You can also have sensual experiences that can seem very confusing and illogical. You can smell, hear screams or cry, feel warm or experience pain. Sometimes you can get disease symptoms and fever that doctors can not diagnose. When sushumna wakes up, you go through a form of depression, anorexia and loneliness. You begin to understand your inner being, your true nature. Materia is experienced as nothing and the body feels as if it were made of air or you can feel as if you are not a part of the body. You can communicate with your surroundings, trees, animals and water. You can start to anticipate things, but usually only boredom, accidents and disasters. You can feel reluctant to do work and it is good if at this stage you can be close to your guru to explain what is happening.

Fine visions and experiences are not always a sushumna or Kundalini awakening. It can still be chakras that open up or experiences of samskaras and archetypes that emerge as a result of the sadhana that one follows. But to roughly sum it up, one can say that a Kundalini awakening always creates more abilities, siddhis. If you slowly begin to understand language better, all of a sudden start to understand complicated things, all of a sudden become good at cooking, all of a sudden get a hearing in music, etc., then a gradual Kundalini awakening is taking place. If you experience temporary sensations and powerful light phenomena or visions, there may be other things that are connected to your chakras.

DIET

When Kundalini is awakened, it is extremely important to follow a proper diet as the food affects the mind and human nature. During awakening, physical changes occur in the body, mainly in the digestive system. The body's internal temperature drops drastically and is much lower compared to the outer body temperature. Metabolism is slow and oxygen consumption decreases. The food must therefore be easy to break down.

The best is cooked food. Crushed wheat, barley, lentils and dal are preferred. Preferably in liquid form. Fatty and heavy foods should be avoided and the amount of protein should be kept to a minimum, as they strain the liver and require a lot of energy to be able to be broken down. When the mind changes, the liver works hard. It is good to increase the carbohydrates in the diet such as rice, potatoes, wheat, and corn. These cause the internal body temperature to increase and do not require much energy to digest.

Spices play a very important role in a Kundalini yogi. Coriander, cumin, anise, black pepper, green pepper, cayenne, mustard seeds, cardamom, cinnamon, etc.

support digestion. They store vital energy and support the internal body tempe-rature.

KRIYA YOGA

Awakening Kundalini is difficult. Most yogic and religious paths are based on a lot of rules that require incredible self-discipline. Rishis in the tantric tradition developed a series of exercises that would be easy to follow and apply, regardless of lifestyle, beliefs or desires. Kriya yoga is seen as one of the most powerful of all tantric exercises and the path that is most suitable for the modern man. The purpose of Kriya yoga is to open up the chakra system, purify the nadis and finally awaken the Kundalini Shakti. Through the various kriyas, Kundalini is aroused gradually. It does not rise suddenly, which would be too difficult to handle.

Unlike other religions and yogic paths that often require strong mind control, in Kriya yoga one should not worry about the mind. Even if you can not concentrate or calm your mind, it does not matter – you develop anyway. Rishis in Kriya yoga believe that control of the mind is not necessary.

"KEEP PRACTICING AND LET THE MIND DO
WHAT IT DOES. IN TIME, CONSCIOUSNESS WILL REACH THE
POINT WHERE THE MIND NO LONGER DISTURBS."

It is not always the fault of the mind that it is anxious or restless. Hormones, indigestion and a weak energy flow in the nervous system can be the cause. One should never blame the mind when it is restless, not even oneself. You are not stupid, bad, unclean or horrible even if you think evil thoughts. Everyone suffers from these, even the most peaceful and devoted. Trying to push back from the mind and thoughts and then see them come back again creates a division and in the worst case causes mental illness. There is no good or evil mind. They are both the same. The mind is nothing but energy. Anger, passion, gratitude and joy are all different forms of the same energy. In Kriya yoga, one tries to utilize this energy without trying to silence or dampen it in any way.

In Kriya yoga, one does not try to concentrate or meditate. Mental control is not the purpose. The mind should flow freely and naturally. Kriya yoga is designed for individuals who find it difficult to sit still and stay focused for a long time. But – everyone should, whether you are tamasic, rajasic or sattvic, practice Hatha yoga as a preparation. A tamasic person needs Hatha yoga to awaken the mind and body. A person who is rajasic needs Hatha yoga to balance the vital and mental energies in the body and mind. A sattvic person needs Hatha yoga to make it easier to awaken Kundalini. In other words, Hatha yoga is for everyone and is a preparation for Kriya yoga. If you have practiced asanas, pranayamas, mudras and bandhas regularly for two years, you are usually ready for Kriya yoga.

There are many Kriyas but twenty of these are the most important and powerful. These twenty are divided into two groups. The first nine are done with open eyes and the remaining eleven are done with closed eyes.

In the first group of exercises, you mustn't close your eyes even if you feel very relaxed and have an easy time turning your mind inward. You can blink, rest, take a break but do not close your eyes.

The first Kriyan is called Vipareeta Karani mudra. It is a method of creating a reverse process in the body. In Hatha Yoga Pradipika and the old tantric texts you can read about this process:

This nectar originates from the moon. As the sun consumes this nectar, the yogi ages. His body collapses and dies. Through regular practice, the yogi should try to reverse this process. The nectar flowing from the moon (Bindu) towards the sun (Manipura) should be returned to the higher centers. When the flow of amrit or nectar can be reversed, it will not be consumed by the sun. It will instead be assimilated by the body."

When the body has been cleansed with Hatha yoga, pranayamas and a pure diet the nectar of the body is assimilated and one experiences a higher mental state. The mind is still and you see and hear everything much clearer.

It is said that one can influence and control the structure and energy of the body and thus evoke peace, dharana, dhyana or samadhi. The various exercises in Kriya yoga such as Vipareeta Karani mudra, Amrit Pan, Khechari mudra, Moola bandha, Maha mudra, and Maha Bheda mudra, regulate the nervous system. The prana in the body is harmonized and balanced. You achieve a state of peace and tranquility without having to fight against the mind. All this by creating a flow of unused and natural chemicals in the body. Amrit is one of them and through Khechari mudra you can make it flow.

Khechari mudra is a simple but very important technique used in most kriyas. By turning the tongue upwards in the palate towards the nasal passage, specific glands and bandages are stimulated, resulting in the amrit starting to flow. One experiences shoonyata, a state of nothingness, being and awareness of everything. Body temperature drops and alpha waves begin to prevail. The mind is completely still.

When you have practiced yoga for a while and have reached the point where you have achieved concentration and a complete inner stillness in body, mind and soul but still feel that there is more to discover, you are ready for Kriya yoga. A calm mind, relaxed body and the right understanding are the results of a spiritual life, however, it is not the ultimate goal. The deeper meaning of yoga is to change the character of the experience, the pattern of the mind and its perception. Man's purpose in practicing yoga has been to expand the mind and release energy. It is tantra and the ultimate goal of Kriya yoga.

THE CHAKRA SYSTEM

THE CHAKRA SYSTEM

In tantra and yoga, the lotus flower is used as a symbol for chakras. Man's spiritual development consists of three important phases: ignorance, striving, or, longing and enlightenment. In the same way, the lotus flower grows through three phases: clay, water and air. It grows in mud (ignorance), grows up through the water to the surface (striving and longing), and finally, it comes up from the water and reaches the air and sunlight (enlightenment).

Each chakra is described as a lotus flower with a specific color and several petals. Each chakra consists of six different aspects:

1. Colour

2. Number of petals

3. Yantra (geometric shape)

4. Beeja mantra (sound/vibration)

5. Animal symbol (represents previous stages of evolution)

6. Higher / eternal being (represents the higher consciousness).

OUR CHAKRA

We have lots of chakras in our body but the most important ones are along our spine. There are also hidden so-called "Secret chakras".
The eight most important chakras in our body are:

MOOLADHARA CHAKRA

The root chakra is located at the base of the spine and is the chakra that vibrates with the lowest frequency, ie. the slowest of our seven chakras. Due to its frequency, its color is dark red and it has four petals. The element associated with this chakra is earth and stands for the most physical and down-to-earth with us.

SWADHISTHANA CHAKRA

The Swadhisthana chakra is located about two centimeters above the tailbone and is the center of our sexuality and reproductive ability. It has six petals, the color orange and its element is water.

MANIPURA CHAKRA

The Manipura chakra is located at the spine at the level of the solar plexus. It has ten petals and the color is yellow. The element fire controls Manipura and it is associated with will, worldly pursuit, ambition and career.

ANAHATA CHAKRA

The Anahatha chakra is located in the spine behind the heart. It has twelve petals and the color is blue or green depending on the tradition you are studying. The element air dominates the chakra and controls our emotions and our relationship with other people. The Anahata chakra is also a symbol of love.

VISHUDDHI CHAKRA

Vishuddhi chakra is located in the neck and has sixteen petals. The color is violet and the element is space (ether). It controls our communication with the environment on different levels.

AJNA CHAKRA

The Ajna chakra is located in the middle of the head at the pineal gland and its contact area is the eyebrow center. It controls our paranormal abilities and siddhis. Also called guru chakra or third eye. It is white and has two petals. It is associated with the mind, reason, intelligence and intuition.

BINDU VISARGA

According to tantra, Bindu visarga is a point located on the back of the head, where the Brahmins usually have their tuft of hair. It represents the crescent with a white drop, which stands for the manifestation of creation, such as consciousness.

SAHASRARA CHAKRA

The chakra is located just above the head and is purple/red. It has a thousand petals and represents pure consciousness. When Kundalini Shakti reaches Sahasrara chakra we become enlightened and according to yoga we enter nirvikalpa samadhi.

KSHETRAM

The exercises in Kundalini yoga usually focus on the trigger point of the chakra, which has its place at the spine. It can be difficult to experience in the beginning and many find it easier to focus on the point of contact on the front of the body called the chakra Kshetram. When we focus on a Kshetram, a sensation is created which then passes via the nerve pathways to the chakra and from there up to the brain. Mooladhara has no contact point, or, Kshetram.

GRANTHIS

We have three granthis (mental knots) in our physical body that are obstacles to Kundalini. These are called Brahma, Vishnu and Rudra. They describe the strength of the Maya, the ignorance and the attraction to material things. Level of consciousness. As an aspirant, one must overcome these obstacles for Kundalini to flow unhindered.

Brahma granthi has its place in the Mooladhara chakra and is associated with the desire for material things, physical satisfaction and selfishness. It is also responsible for tamas – negativity, lethargy and ignorance.

Vishnu granthi has its place in the Anahata chakra and is associated with emotional desires, depending on people and inner mental visions. It is linked to rajas and has tendencies toward passion, ambition and determination.

Rudra granthi rules over the Ajna chakra. It is associated with the desire for Siddhis, mental phenomena and the image of ourselves as individuals.

THE EVOLUTION THROUGH THE CHAKRANA

Human evolution as individuals and as a race is a journey through our chakras. Mooladhara is the base and Sahasrara is the very goal or end of evolution.

In animals, Mooladhara is the highest chakra. It is their Sahasrara. Until Mooladhara, evolution takes place by itself, it is under the control of nature. When Kundalini reaches Mooladhara, evolution no longer happens automatically. Man is no longer subordinate to the laws of nature. Man is aware of time and space. Man has an ego, he can think, is aware that he is thinking and he knows that he is aware that he is thinking. Without the ego, there is no double consciousness. Animals do not have a double consciousness. Man thus has a higher consciousness and must therefore also work to develop it. Therefore, it is said that Kundalini lies dormant in Mooladhara until it is awakened for further development.

Awakening Kundalini is a process. It may wake up to return to Mooladhara several times. When it finally reaches the Manipura chakra in a steady state, it will not turn again. What can happen is that it can get stuck in a chakra if there are blockages or if the sushumna is not open. Kundalini can remain in a chakra for several years or even a lifetime.

Before starting to practice Kundalini yoga, it is important to find out in which chakra Kundalini is located. The easiest way to do this is to focus on each chakra individually for fifteen minutes over fifteen days. You will notice which chakra is easiest to experience and stay focused on. Here is Kundalini Shakti.

Awakening our chakras plays an important role in human evolution. It has nothing to do with mystery or anything occult. When the chakras are awakened, our consciousness and our mind change. This affects our daily lives as our mind is what controls how we act in different situations, relationships and emotions.

Today, many children are born with open chakras and Kundalini. When these children grow up, they behave differently. Our modern society often sees these differences as something abnormal and the result is often mental health care or similar. Going through conflicts within family and work is a common pheno-menon, but when the mind and consciousness begin to expand, one becomes extremely sensitive to everything that happens in the mind, family, colleagues and society. You can not overlook something that happens in life. It is not seen as normal by most people but it is a natural consequence of the chakra being awakened. Consciousness becomes very receptive when the frequency of the mind changes.

Love, devotion, charity, etc. are all expressions of a mind affected by the chakra in balance. This is the reason why so much emphasis is placed on awakening the Anahata chakra, or, the heart chakra. All chakras are of course important to open up and all have different qualities, but you can see that in most ancient scriptures put extra emphasis on awakening the Anahata, Ajna and Mooladha-ra chakra. When Anahata is awakened, we get a deeper relationship with our family and all individuals.

When the chakras are opened, the mind changes automatically. Values change and love and relationships change character. Disappointments and feelings of frustration are balanced, which leads to a better attitude toward ourselves and life.

PREPARATIONS FOR KRIYA YOGA

Kriya yoga is considered by many to be the most effective method of developing human consciousness. These exercises are said to be those that Shiva gave to his wife, Parvati. Kriyas are relatively simple and not too powerful for the average person to perform.

Before you start practicing Kriya yoga, it is important that you can feel the chakras in the body, both mentally and physically, and be able to locate its Kshetram. One should also know two mental passages in the body "arohan" and "awarohan".

To develop in Kundalini yoga and preparation for Kriya yoga, it is important to be well acquainted with the following techniques:

Vipareeta karani asana
Ujjayi pranayama
Siddhasana / Siddha yoni asana
Unmani mudra
Khechari mudra
Ajapa Japa
Utthanpadasana
Shambhavi mudra
Moola bandha
Nasikagra drishti
Uddiyana bandha
Jalandhara bandha
Bhadrasana
Padmasana
Shanmuki mudra
Varjoli / Sahajoli mudra

IDA AND PINGALA

Yogis have described that man has three main flows of energy in the body. Ida, pingala and sushumna nadi. These can be roughly translated as mind, body and spirit. Sushumna is the result of a balanced and harmonious flow between ida and pingala.

Nadis are flows of energy that move throughout our bodies. All the thousands of nadis that flow in the body are connected to the ida and pingala nadi that move along the spine. Every cell in our body, organ, brain and mind is linked on a mental and physical level, which allows us to speak, think and act in a balanced and correct way. Ida and pingala nadi are the ones who control the balance between them. By affecting a part of the system, the whole system is affected.

This is how asanas, pranayamas, meditation and the whole yogic system work. Yoga thus affects the entire system of nadis in our body.

Yogis and scientists have come to the same result, albeit with different ways of describing it. Man has two main modes through which he functions. The pattern of the brain is based on ida and pingala nadi, consciousness or knowledge, action or physical energy. We can see ida and pingala nadis functions in the three main parts of the nervous system.

A sensory-motor nervous system is where all electrical activity in the body moves within two paths through the body. Into the brain (afferent), ida and out through the brain (efferent), pingala.

The autonomic nervous system is divided into the outward, stress management, energy utilization, pingala dominant, sympathetic nervous system and inward, relaxed, energy saving, ida dominant parasympathetic nervous system.

Central nervous system which consists of the brain and spine and which controls the two preceding parts of the nervous system.

What the yogic techniques are based on is the knowledge of our nadis and chakras. The physical experience of these is that you can also experience on a physical level through the different parts of the nervous system. The influence of the nervous system on our physical body describes the importance of balancing and harmonizing the flow between ida, pingala and sushumna nadi.

THE IMPORTANCE OF PREPARATION, EXERCISE AND NOT TAKING WATER OVER YOUR HEAD

As a beginner in yoga and full of desire and inspiration, it is easy to get water over your head. Yoga is a process in which the body and mind are prepared for more advanced techniques. It's like running. If you have run several marathons, you may need to run longer stretches to feel that the training gives something.

This does not mean that you as a new runner do not get the benefits out of running three kilometers. This is exactly how yoga works.

When you have practiced Hatha yoga for a few years and feel comfortable in the positions with all the locks and postures and master the breathing exercises, you can move on with the most advanced tantric techniques. Then they will not feel too complicated and you will have a consciousness that allows you to enjoy the effects of your practice without it becoming too much. If something feels too complicated, go back one step instead. Everything comes to you when you are ready. Hurry slowly.

"YOU EXPERIENCE ALL THE POWER
IN THE COSMOS AND ON EARTH,
IN YOURSELF AND AROUND.
EVERYTHING YOU WANT IS POSSIBLE
BECAUSE ALL POWER IS YOURS!"

CHAKRANA
INDEX

AJNA CHAKRA

ALSO CALLED THE THIRD EYE

TANMATRA *(a sensory experience):* Sense.

JNANENDRIYA *(sense organ):* Sense.

KARMENDRIYA *(body of action):* Sense.

TATTWA *(element):* Sense.

BIJA MANTRA: *Om.*

TATTWA SYMBOL: *Picture of the mantra Om.*

YOGA TYPE: *Jnana, Raja and Mantra yoga (Sattvic).*

LOTUS (PADMA): *White, silver or smoky with two petals.*

AJNA CHAKRA *(third eye) is associated with the mind, reason, intelligence and intuition. It is also the center through which two people through the mind – on a deeper level, are in contact with each other. For example, the contact between guru (teacher/master) and student/disciple.*

Direct concentration on the Ajna chakra is very difficult and therefore one focuses on tantra and yoga in the middle of the eyebrow center (which is the Kshetram of the Ajna chakra). This point is called bhrumadhya (bhru- refers to eyebrows and madhya refers to the center), and lies between the eyebrows at the place where Indian ladies put a red dot and Pandits and Brahmins put a mark. This eyebrow center can be touched by various techniques.

Ajna and Mooladhara chakras are closely related, and awakening in one of these helps to awaken the others. Ideally, Ajna should be awakened to some extent before Mooladhara to prepare the mind for all the hidden memories and impressions that come to the surface as we practice chakra awakening. But the awakening in Mooladhara will also help to further awaken Ajna. The best way to bring about the awakening of Ajna is moola bandha and ashwini mudra, which are specific to Mooladhara.

It should also be mentioned that the Ajna chakra and the pineal gland are the same. Just like the pituitary gland is the physical aspect of Sahasrara. The pituitary gland and the pineal gland are intimately connected, as are the Ajna and Sahasrara. We can say that Ajna is the gateway to the Sahasrara chakra. If Ajna is awakened and works, then all experiences in Sahasrara happen as well.

The pineal gland acts as a lock for the pituitary gland. As long as the pineal gland is healthy, the pituitary gland works on a deeper, spiritual level. But for most of us, the pineal gland stops developing when we turn eight, nine or ten years old. This is when the pituitary gland begins to function and secrete various hormones that stimulate our sexual consciousness, our sensuality and worldly person. At this time, we started to lose touch with our spiritual heritage. However, through various yogic techniques, such as trataka and shambhavi mudra, it is possible to restore or maintain the health of the pineal gland. The pineal gland and Ajna chakra have a special significance in esoteric yoga and tantra. It is the place where siddhis (occult/magical) abilities are manifested.

The "third eye" is a mysterious and esoteric concept that can refer to Ajna chakra in various spiritual traditions from the East and West. It is also said to be a door that leads into inner worlds and stages of higher consciousness. In tantra and yoga, the "third eye" can symbolize enlightenment or the development of mental images with deeply spiritual or psychological meanings. The "third eye" is often associated with siddhis such as revelations, clairvoyance (which also includes

The Chakranas
Colour No. of Petals Yantra
Action Element & Bija mantra

Sahasrara chakra – I understand
dark red, 1000 petals. Aum, Shiva

Ajna chakra	Third Eye
White, 2 Petals	I see
Pyramid	Moon Aum
Vishuddhi c.	I talk
Purple 16 petals	Space Element
Cirkel with Space	mantra Ham
Anahata chakra.	I love
Blue, 12 petals	Air element
Blue Davidstar	mantra Yam
Manipura chakra	I do
Yellow, 10 petals	Fire element
Red triangel	mantra Ram
Swadhisthana c.	I feel
Orange, 10 petals	Water element
Half moon	mantra Vam

Mooladhara chakra – I am
Red 4 petals. Bija mantra Lam
Earth element, Yellow square

experiences. A person who is considered to have developed an ability to use his
"third eye" is called a Siddha in yoga, and is referred to as a person who has
developed siddhis.

"THE PINEAL GLAND AND THE DMT MOLECULE - THE THIRD EYE ... THERE MAY BE A WAY FOR THE BRAIN TO TAKE US TO A HIGHER PLANE OF EXISTENCE, WHERE WE CAN UNDERSTAND THE WORLD AND OUR RELATIONSHIPS TO THINGS AND PEOPLE ON A DEEPER LEVEL AND WHERE WE CAN ULTIMATELY CREATE A DEEPER MEANING FOR OURSELVES AND OUR WORLD. THERE IS A SPIRITUAL PART OF THE BRAIN - IT IS A PART THAT WE CAN ALL HAVE ACCESS TO AND IS SOMETHING THAT WE ALL CAN ACCOMPLISH."

(ANDREW NEWBERG - BRAIN RESEARCHER)

MOOLADHARA CHAKRA

TANMATRA *(a sensory experience): Smell.*

JNANENDRIYA *(sense organ): Nose.*

KARMENDRIYA *(organ of action): Anus.*

TATTWA *(element): Prithvi (earth).*

BIJA MANTRA: *Lam.*

TATTWA SYMBOL: *Yellow square.*

ANIMALS: *Elephant.*

YOGA TYPE: *Tantra and Hatha yoga (counteracts tamas/inertia).*

LOTUS (PADMA): *Red lotus with four petals.*

MOOLADHARA CHAKRA

Moola means root. A triangular space in the middle of the body at a point between the genitals and anus for men and at the cervix for women. Mooladhara is associated with personal security in both thought and action. At this level, the individual focuses mainly on obtaining food and shelter and securing his reproduction. She surrounds herself with material things, money, family and friends to create personal security.

In the middle of Mooladhara, one usually imagines a black swayambhu linga (a symbol of male power, Shiva). Around this, the serpent Kundalini (Shakti, the mother of all prana in the human body) winds three and a half turns – dozing in anticipation of its awakening, as it ascends through sushumna nadi to unite with Shiva in Sahasrara padma in the moment of enlightenment. This can only happen when the individual's spiritual development has reached the necessary maturity.

MOOLADHARA'S IMPACT ON OUR DIFFERENT BODIES

IN ANNAMAYA KOSHA *(physical body).*
Reproductive organs, perineum, uterine tube.

IN PRANAMAYA KOSHA *(energy body).*
Apana vayu.

IN MANOMAYA KOSHA *(body of thought).*
Security, ownership, safety, survival.

MOOLADHARA IN DIFFERENT STAGES OF GUNAS

Creation and its energy consist of three gunas, fundamental properties or tendencies: Sattva, rajas and tamas. These three gunas act and react incessantly with each other. The world of phenomena is composed of different combinations of these three gunas. Tamas stands for inertia, rajas for movement and sattva for balance. When Mooladhara is in balance and sattvic, we are safe and secure in ourselves and the world. When Mooladhara is out of balance and is tamasic, we experience boundless fear. We are in a deep psychosis. As the balance becomes more rajasic, our condition changes as shown below. By identifying one's state with the right degree of imbalance/balance in the various chakras, the yogi believes that he can alleviate and dissolve negative states.

TAMAS: *Horror.*

TAMAS / RAJAS: *Anxiety, worries.*

RAJAS / TAMAS: *Greed, self-confidence.*

RAJAS: *Collector.*

RAJAS / SATTVA: *Generosity.*

SATTVA / RAJAS: *Property for good cause.*

SATTVA: *Safe in the physical world.*

ENLIGHTENED: *Unity with the absolute*

SWADHISTHANA CHAKRA

TANMATRA *(a sensory experience): Taste.*

JNANENDRIYA *(sense organ): Tongue.*

KARMENDRIYA *(organ of action): Genitals.*

TATTWA *(element): Apas (water).*

BIJA MANTRA: *Vam.*

TATTWA SYMBOL: *White crescent.*

ANIMALS: *Crocodile.*

YOGA TYPE: *Tantra and Hatha yoga (counteracts tamas/inertia).*

LOTUS (PADMA): *Orange lotus with six petals.*

SWADHISTHANA CHAKRA *(pleasure, lust)*
The chakra sits at the base of the spine just inside the lower tailbone and at the height of the genitals. Chakra is associated with sensory experiences. One strives to achieve sensory enjoyment through e.g. food, drinks, sex, etc. You value everything in terms of the enjoyment you can thereby achieve. The difference from the Mooladhara chakra is that here we strive for the pleasure of the mind itself, rather than for satisfying basic needs.

It is said that most people in the world primarily act and are motivated at this level. Swadhisthana chakra is also usually associated with the unconscious. It is said that coexistence – traces or patterns created in the unconscious of the experiences we make and the actions we perform have their place in this chakra. Samskaras eventually form the basis of the individual's karma. Most of these co-habitants are displaced from consciousness or can be even repressed. Therefore, the Swadhisthana chakra is often associated with desires, urges, and fears over which we have no control.

THE IMPACT OF SWADHISTHANA ON OUR DIFFERENT BODIES

ANNAMAYA KOSHA *(physical body): Genitals, urination.*

PRANAMAYA KOSHA *(energy body): Apana vayu.*

MANOMAYA KOSHA *(body of thought): Satisfaction, pleasure, sex (from pleasure to addiction).*

SWADHISTHANA IN DIFFERENT STAGES OF GUNAS

TAMAS: *Depression.*

TAMAS / RAJAS: *Bitterness, the feeling of being rejected.*

RAJAS / TAMAS: *Desire, sexual exploitation.*

RAJAS: *Seeking pleasure, sexual conquests.*

RAJAS / SATTVA: *Humor, caring sexuality with love.*

SATTVA / RAJAS: *Happily satisfied.*

SATTVA: *Bubbly happy.*

ENLIGHTENED: *Ananda, happiness "bliss".*

MANIPURA CHAKRA

TANMATRA *(a sensory experience): Vision.*

JNANENDRIYA *(sensory organs): Eyes.*

KARMENDRIYA *(organ of action): Feet.*

TATTWA *(element): Agni (fire).*

BIJA MANTRA: *Ram.*

TATTWA SYMBOL: *Red inverted triangle.*

ANIMALS: *Aries.*

YOGA TYPE: *Karma yoga (counteracts rajas/mobility).*

LOTUS (PADMA): *Yellow lotus with ten petals.*

MANIPURA *(seat of the jewel)*
The chakra is located in the spine at the level of the navel. It is associated with will, worldly pursuit, ambition and career. From the energy of manipulation, man grows as a social and self-conscious being. She cultivates material desires, such as owning and mastering, power, prestige and usefulness. But also selfless-ness, social balance and prosperity.

Manipura's energy is outward and active, a vital energy that provides the power to act and the power to change oneself and one's surroundings. Sometimes this happens with a selfish attitude where other people are seen as a means to achieve their ambition, but here also the first expressions of a growing self-awa-

reness begin to take shape in man. The ego is still dominant but the first traces of a genuine, spiritual pursuit are manifested at this level. One begins to seriously question one's existence and one's motives.

THE IMPACT OF MANIPURA ON OUR DIFFERENT BODIES

ANNAMAYA KOSHA *(physical body): Solar Plexus, digestion.*

PRANAMAYA KOSHA *(energy body): Samana vayu.*

MANOMAYA KOSHA *(body of thought): Power, action, self-confidence and striving.*

MANIPURA IN DIFFERENT STAGES OF GUNAS

TAMAS: *Inability to act.*

TAMAS / RAJAS: *Guilt over non-actions, low self-esteem.*

RAJAS / TAMAS: *Frustration over one's inability.*

RAJAS: *Active, brave.*

RAJAS / SATTVA: *Anxious, ready to act.*

SATTVA / RAJAS: *Karma yoga at an intermediate level.*

SATTVA: *Things happen as if by miracle.*

ENLIGHTENED: *Omnipotent.*

ANAHATA CHAKRA

TANMATRA *(a sensory experience): Feeling.*

JNANENDRIYA *(sense organ): Skin.*

KARMENDRIYA *(body of action): Hands.*

TATTWA *(element): Vayu (air).*

BIJA MANTRA: *Yam.*

TATTWA SYMBOL: *Blue hexagram.*

ANIMALS: *Black antelope.*

YOGA TYPE: *Bhakti and Karma yoga (counteracts rajas/mobility).*

LOTUS (PADMA): *Blue or green lotus with twelve petals.*

ANAHATA *(unspoken "sound", the origin of all mantras). Anahata sits in the spine at the height of the heart. Its energy is associated with love, hate, joy and sorrow as well as with the beauty experience. Chakra is strongly associated with our relationships with others around us.*

At this level, the individual often begins to love everything and everyone unconditionally. You learn to ignore the faults and shortcomings of others and take them for what they are. Anahata also stands for aesthetic discernment and artistic creation. The energy is expressed here in the form of creativity regardless of which area you are active in. At this level, man leaves the material world to cultivate higher values.

THE INFLUENCE OF ANAHATA IN OUR DIFFERENT BODIES

ANNAMAYA KOSHA *(physical body): Heart, lungs.*

PRANAMAYA KOSHA *(energy body): Vyana vayu.*

MANOMAYA KOSHA *(body of thought): Love, compassion, acceptance and tolerance.*

ANAHATHA IN DIFFERENT STAGES OF GUNAS

TAMAS: *Apathy.*

TAMAS / RAJAS: *Fraud, treason.*

RAJAS / TAMAS: *Avoid intimacy.*

RAJAS: *Love under certain conditions.*

RAJAS / SATTVA: *Care about others.*

SATTVA / RAJAS: *Love and compassion.*

SATTVA: *Is love.*

ENLIGHTENED: *Cosmic love.*

VISHUDDHI CHAKRA

TANMATRA *(a sensory experience):* Sound.

JNANENDRIYA *(sensory organs):* Ears.

KARMENDRIYA *(body of action):* Body of speech.

TATTWA *(element):* Akasha (space).

BIJA MANTRA: *Ham.*

TATTWA SYMBOL: *White and black circle.*

ANIMALS: *White elephant.*

YOGA TYPE: *Jnana, Raja and Mantra yoga (sattvic)*

LOTUS (PADMA): *Violet lotus with sixteen petals.*

VISHUDDHI (purity).

The chakra sits in the neck behind the larynx and is associated with an attitude of independence (vairagya), where both pleasant and unpleasant aspects of human life are seen and accepted as rewarding experiences. The world appears as a place full of harmony and perfection. Everything you experience, good or bad, is seen as part of a whole that helps to remove personal problems, locks and limitations and raise the level of consciousness. This attitude leads to discernment (viveka).

Vishuddhi is also associated with expression, communication in general and the spoken word in particular.

THE IMPACT OF VISHUDDHI ON OUR DIFFERENT BODIES

ANNAMAYA KOSHA *(physical body): The thyroid gland, parathyroid gland, trachea and esophagus.*

PRANAMAYA KOSHA *(energy body): Udana vayu.*

MANOMAYA KOSHA *(body of thought): Communication.*

VISHUDDHI IN DIFFERENT STAGES OF GUNAS

TAMAS: *Isolated.*

TAMAS / RAJAS: *Limited contact / communication.*

RAJAS / TAMAS: *Complaining/whining.*

RAJAS: *Pretty good communicator.*

RAJAS / SATTVA: *Eloquent.*

SATTVA / RAJAS: *Persuader, non-violent communication.*

SATTVA: *True communication.*

ENLIGHTENED: *Cosmic communication.*

BINDU VISARGA

Bindu visarga is located on top of the back of the head. Many claims that one can not find Bindu in the physical body but that it can only be experienced via nada, ie. via its vibration or sound. It is not a chakra in the ordinary sense.

Through techniques like moorcha pranayama and vajroli / sahajoli mudra we can develop the experience of nada and through techniques like bhramari pranayama and shanmukhi mudra we can follow nada to its source – Bindu.

There is a close relationship between the Swadhisthana chakra and the Bindu. This is because Bindu is the point where the vibration and sound of the individual creation are first manifested, and Swadhisthana is the center of creation in the form of sexual reproduction. Through Swadhisthana, our physical desire for union with the cosmic consciousness is expressed. Sperm and menstruation are physical expressions of the drops of amrit – the nectar drops of creation or secretions that drip from the Bindu and are burned in the Manipura chakra via the Vishuddhi chakra. The drops control the creation process and the body's aging.

It is commonly believed that there is no Kshetram – contact point for Bindu visarga.

SAHASRARA CHAKRA

The chakra is located just above the head and is purple/red. It has a thousand petals and represents pure consciousness. When Kundalini Shakti reaches Sahasrara chakra we become enlightened and according to yoga we enter nirvikalpa samadhi.

The function of the Sahasrara is to provide us with other levels of consciousness, which may make us realize that "we are one" and that "everything is one". It is through the crown chakra that we experience union with God and with the supernatural. The Crown chakra is what is called "pure consciousness".

When one reaches a higher level of consciousness in this chakra, all thinking is released. Here lay the answers to all our questions, the absolute truth that we all dream of getting answers to, and where we find total freedom – We become enlightened.

LESSON NO. 4

LONG SHAVASANA – DEAD MAN'S POSTURE/RELAXATION.

PRANAYAMA – YOGIC BREATHING.

SUPTA PAWANMUKTASANA – THE LEG LOCK.

SURYA NAMASKARA – SUN SALUTATION WITHOUT BREATHING.

TRIKONASANA – THE TRIANGLE STAND.

SHAVASANA – DEAD MAN'S POSTURE.

SHAVA UDARAKARSHANASANA – THE UNIVERSAL POSITION.

SHAVASANA – DEAD MAN'S POSTURE.

BHUJANGASANA – THE COBRA.

SHASHANK ASANA – THE HARE.

SHAVASANA – DEAD MAN'S POSTURE.

YOGA NIDRA – DEEP RELAXATION.

KAYA STHAIRYAM & AJAPA JAPA – STEP 1 – MEDITATION.

END WITH – HARI OM TAT SAT, 3 TIMES.

THEN – OM SRI DURGAYAI NAMAH, 1 TIME.

INSTRUCTIONS FOR ASANAS LESSON NO. 4

LONG SHAVASANA – DEAD MAN'S POSTURE/RELAXATION.

Execution: See module 1.

PRANAYAMA – YOGIC BREATHING.

Execution: See modules 1 & 2.

SUPTA PAWANMUKTASANA – THE LEG LOCK.

Execution: See modules 1 & 2.

SURYA NAMASKARA – SUN SALUTATION WITHOUT BREATHING.

Execution: See module 3.

TRIKONASANA – THE TRIANGLE STAND.

Execution: Stand with your feet wide apart on the long side of the mat. Keep your legs straight throughout the exercise. Turn the front foot so that it points straight ahead in line with the front arm. Make sure the front foot is in a straight line with the back foot. Lift the rear arm straight up and look down at the front. Follow it with your eyes as it goes down along the calf. When your buttocks start to push backward, you have gone down too far. Your body should be completely straight. Your behind should be in line with your shoulders. Then look up at the backhand and turn the palm in the same direction as the tip of the nose. Stand in the position for a few minutes and then continue with the other side.

SHAVASANA – DEAD MAN'S POSTURE.

Execution: See module no. 1 & 2.

SHAVA UDARAKARSHANASANA – THE UNIVERSAL POSITION.

Execution: See modules 1 & 2.

BHUJANGASANA – THE COBRA.

Execution: See module 2.

SHASHANKASANA - THE HARE.

Execution: See modules 1 & 2.

YOGA NIDRA – DEEP RELAXATION.

Execution: See module 3.

KAYA STHAIRYAM & AJAPA JAPA – STEP 2 – MEDITATION.

Execution: See module 3.

MANIPURA CHAKRA

To practice regularly for a month.

Chakra and kshetram localization/activation and purification through uddiyana bandha/belly lock with Ram chanting. Inhale and hold your breath as you inhale using the diaphragm and practice the stomach lock/uddiyana bandha. Experience the pulsation from the chakra and visualize the color while you say Ram quietly to yourself. You can also visualize the yantra.

Bhastrika & kapalbhati with uddiyana bandha. Inhale and expand your stomach, exhale and contract – bhastrika, practice this for about 30 rounds and then hold your breath out and lean forward on straight arms with your hands on your knees and practice stomach locks. The same technique with kapalbhati but now you put all the focus on the exhalation and let the inhalation take care of itself.

Union with prana and apana vayu. Sit in a meditation position and experience how prana vayu moves down to the navel and unites with apana vayu which moves up from the anus to the navel on inhalation. Exhale and the energy currents turn and move up and down the body. Continue for about five minutes.

KNOWLEDGE TEST MODULE 4

ANSWER AS FULLY AS YOU CAN, THEN CHECK IF YOU ANSWERED CORRECTLY. PRACTICE UNTIL YOU KNOW THE ANSWERS BY HEART.

1. DESCRIBE KUNDALINI SHAKTI.

2. EXPLAIN THE METHODS.

3. DESCRIBE KRIYA YOGA.

4. WHAT IS THE CHAKRA SYSTEM?

5. DESCRIBE THE EVOLUTION THROUGH THE CHAKRANA.

6. TALK ABOUT POTENTIAL RISKS WITH A KUNDALINI AWAKENING.

7. WHY IS IT IMPORTANT TO TAKE THINGS SLOWLY IN YOGA?

8. EXPLAIN HOW TO EXPERIENCE THE AWAKENING.

9. DESCRIBE MANIPURA CHAKRA, ITS ELEMENT, YANTRA, COLOR, NUMBER OF CROWNS AND PROPERTIES.

10. DESCRIBE SOME POWERFUL EXERCISES TO ACTIVATE, CLEAN AND BALANCE MANIPURA CHAKRA.

MODULE 5

KARMA, BHAKTI & JNANA YOGA. WE STUDY YOGA FROM A HINDU PERSPECTIVE

We study Karma, Bhakti and Jnana yoga and its context. We study the Anahata chakra and practice our exercises to cleanse, balance and activate the chakra. We continue to practice in the role of yoga teacher with lesson no. 5 of 8.

Knowledge test: Answer the questions related to module 5. Practice lesson no. 5 with at least 1 participant and humbly accept feedback from them. Ask questions afterward – how was the pace, did you keep to time, did you speak loudly enough, and how well did you understand the exercises?

KARMA, BHAKTI & JNANA YOGA

HINDUISM

Hinduism differs from other religions in that it can be described as a collective name for a host of religious denominations that lack a common core. Most Hindus see Hinduism as a set of ritual acts, something practiced. But Hinduism is also a tradition that carries a large set of knowledge – it is the religion that has the largest number of sacred texts.

In Hinduism, humans are perceived as thinking, biological and social beings characterized by people's different interests and aptitudes for things. They worship different gods, read different texts, follow different teaching systems and gurus, and visit different temples. This view is the basis for the hierarchical system applied in Hinduism but also the tolerance that exists for each other's differences and diversity.

Diversity expresses the process of change and development that matter, Prakriti, undergoes. Purusha, on the other hand, is what all individuals have in common – the unchanging self, the atman, as the samkhya philosophy describes.

Samkhya and yoga both belong to the philosophical system of Hinduism. The purpose of the systems is to guide man towards moksha, or freedom from the cycle of rebirth. Moksha is considered to be the fourth and final goal in a person's life.

The six philosophical systems are arranged in doctrinal pairs as follows:
Nyaya – logic
Vaisheshika – atomic

Samkhya – cosmic principle
Yoga – yoga

Purva-Mimamsa (Vedanta) – ritual

Uttara-Mimamsa (Vedanta) – theological

The belief, within these systems, of a person's ability to be liberated, differs from the bhakti-oriented theistic Vedan schools, whose adherents believe that a person is dependent on the grace of God to be free from the cycle of rebirth.

Samkhya and yoga are described together in many Hindu texts, indicating an early connection to each other.

The Katha, Svetasvatara and Maitri Upanishads describe yogic exercises and samkhya together. In the Katha Upanishad, yoga is used as a means of meditation. Yoga and samkhya are also mentioned in close connection in the Mahabharata. Here, the goal of yoga is described as the realization of the atman (the self) and brahman (matter).

The Bhagavad Gita, which is part of the Mahabharata, describes yoga in three different ways – Jnana, Karma and Bhakti yoga. Krishna is seen here as the master of yoga.

The Yoga Sutras of Patanjali, an important text in Hinduism, and the most important work of classical yoga, have become and serve as a basic description of it. Here too, samkhya plays a central role. Even yoga traditions that do not share the same view of the ultimate reality have embraced the Yoga Sutras, which describe them logically and coherently. In the Yoga Sutras, yoga is described as the cessation of the activities of the mind, what we today call meditation.

DHARMA

A central concept in Hinduism is dharma, likened to duty, law, rightness and firmness. Many Hindus today call their religion Sanatana dharma (the eternal dharma). Dharma is the eternal order, and in the oldest scriptures, it refers to the various rituals and duties performed to maintain social and cosmic order.

Dharma is based on the notion that humans maintain the universe through their actions. These actions are covered by various rituals, civil and criminal law, stages of life, pilgrimages, sacrifices, etc. Dharma is used to structure society and the life of the individual. It plays a significant role in the caste systems applied in Hindu society. Following one's dharma should lead to a better rebirth and be a path to ultimate salvation.

TRADITIONS

The core tradition of Hinduism is Brahmanical: the most dominant and widespread tradition in India. Men in the tradition are authoritarian. The Vedic texts play a central role and are seen as revelations. Within the tradition are the priesthood, a sacred language (Sanskrit) and the perception of a sacred social order. Rituals are performed in temples and ceremonies in the home. Various Hindu deities are worshipped, such as Shiva, Vishnu, Rama, Krishna, Durga, Kali and Ganesha. Pilgrimages, festivals, rules about food and cleanliness are also important.

The other major focus is organizations, where the focus is usually on moksha (salvation). These usually have a founder and some are more ritually oriented (Sri Vishnuism and Sri Vidya), while others function as organizations for ascetics (Vishnuite: Ramanandi and Nada; or Shivaite: Natha and Aghori). They are often bearers of different yoga traditions and men from the Brahmin class are often seen as leaders of these groups.

The guru movements also belong to this tradition; these often have to compete for followers. Many have also succeeded in communicating their teachings internationally such as Maharishi Mahesh Yogi (Transcendental Meditation) and A.C. Bhaktivedanta Swami Prabhupada (International Society for Krishna Consciousness).

A third focus is the village and tribe-based traditions of India. Priests in this tradition are not from the Brahmin class and gods who have a local connection are worshipped. The Brahmin core tradition sees these practices as unclean, which has led to a tense relationship.

VISHNUISM, SHIVAISM AND SHAKTISM

Sacrifice rituals were a central part of the Brahmanic tradition, but became less important as the ascetic ideology emerged. Knowledge and renunciation became more important than being freed from the cycle of rebirth. Many of the gods who were important in the Vedic sacrificial tradition fell away, while Shiva and Vishnu remain important. Groups sprang up where one of these gods was worshipped, laying the foundation for Hinduism as a religion. The ritual worship of gods (puja) that then arose competed with the sacrificial culture (yajna).

Seventy percent of Hindus worship Vishnu or one of his avatars, such as Rama or Krishna. Vishnu's task is to sustain the world. In the form of Krishna, he evokes feelings of love and care. In the form of Rama, he symbolizes the world order, dharma and the dutiful man. Worship and devotion to a personal god is what characterizes Vishnuism, but there are also organizations for ascetics and some groups have taken up some of tantrism and instead worship a goddess such as Lakshmi.

Twenty-eight percent of Hindus worship Shiva and his family members, his wife Parvati and their sons Ganesha and Skanda. Shiva is a great yogi and a friendly god but also has sides where he appears dangerous, destructive and terrible. Shivaism is common in the Himalayan region and is largely yogic. Some Hindu ascetics also worship him.

The 13th to 16th centuries were a great time for Shivaite ascetics and Natha yogis in northern India. They practiced hatha yoga and various tantric rituals. Gorakhnatha is the most famous Natha yogi. He was a student of Matsyendra-natha, who himself was a disciple of Shiva. Through Hatha yoga, one could stop the decay of the body and activate Kundalini Shakti, to create an immortal body that would lead to the Shiva state. According to Natha yogis, only Hatha yoga could lead to this condition; other religious paths were considered unnecessary.

About two percent of Hindus follow Shaktism and worship the goddess Shakti, the female power of the supreme divine principle. She is seen as the ultimate reality (brahman), the creative power (Shakti), the matter in creation (Prakriti), the one who hides (maya) and the savior. Shaktism has evolved from Shivaism. Many female figures were found during the excavations in the Indus Valley, although it is unclear what they represented. It was not until the seventh century AD, that Shaktism was mentioned in the written traditions.

Female ideology also plays a central role in tantrism, whose concept is based on the belief that our external environment and our bodies consist of both female and male aspects, and that salvation comes through uniting this polarity. To achieve tantric salvation (sadhana), mantras, mudras, nyasa and puja are used. Tantrism combines Jnana and Karma yoga. Knowledge is what ultimately saves a person and action is what gives them experience of the ultimate reality. Kundalini yoga was developed as a separate branch of yoga within tantrism and is based on the goddess ideology of tantrism and Shaktism. The path of tantrism is the most effective for the world we live in today, the Kali era. Old techniques are more difficult to apply.

HINDUISM AND YOGA

In the 1920s, archaeological excavations were made along the Indus River and uncovered the remains of two large cities, Mohenjo Daro and Harappa. Both yoga and Hinduism most likely originate from this era, when the Indus and Saraswati civilizations existed.

The excavations also uncovered fall stones, which are an important symbol of the god Shiva, and signets, one of which depicted a person with animal horns sitting in a meditation position surrounded by four animals. Shiva is often called the master of animals, which may indicate that he was already being worshipped when the Indus culture flourished between 5,000 and 3,000 BC. Shiva is called the great yogi, which indicates that yoga's origins were from this time.

Modern technology has helped to establish that the river Saraswati dried up sometime during the 30th century BC. In the Rigveda, the river Saraswati is praised, suggesting this sacred text must have come into being earlier. Yoga is mentioned in the Rigveda, indicating that it too probably originated before the 30th century BC.

Yoga plays a central role in Hinduism and is used as a method of physical and mental discipline as well as to achieve spiritual salvation. It is the part of Hinduism that most people have experienced – both Hindus and non-Hindus. The original goal of yoga in the Hindu tradition is to reach salvation or enlightenment with the help of the body, using various physical and mental techniques. In the West, yoga has mostly been used to strengthen the body and find peace. Like Hinduism, yoga is also pluralistic, which means that there are many different types of physical and mental exercises depending on which tradition you choose.

Traditions can define the concept of yoga in different ways. The most common translation among Hindus is "union", which refers to a union between body and soul. In the Patanjali Yoga Sutras, one of the most important texts in yoga, it is defined as yoga chitta vritti nirodhah, or cessation of the activities of the mind.

Within the yoga traditions, the term yoga has five main meanings:

1. A disciplined method of achieving a goal.
2. A technique for controlling the body.
3. A name for one of the six philosophical systems of Hinduism.
4. In combination with other words such as Hatha, mantra and laya, yoga refers to traditions that have focused on specific yoga techniques.
5. Objectives for the practice of yoga.

Central to any tradition is breathing and breath control. Holding the breath is considered in the Brahmanic tradition as a ritual act. Atharvaveda tells of breathing and its connection to the body's energies. The Chandogya Upanishad describes five different types of breathing, the inner sound and the nadis.

YOGA AND BUDDHISM

Buddhism has its roots in Indian yoga and was from its beginning a form of yoga. The Buddha himself was taught by yoga teachers and his experiences became the basis of the Buddhist meditation doctrine. Buddhist yoga and Hindu yoga are thus closely related and may have influenced each other for many hundreds of years. Concepts such as nirodha/nirvana (cessation) and dukkha (suffering) are common to both traditions. The Buddhist eight-fold path and Indian eight-fold yoga have many similarities. The big difference is that in Indian yoga the body and breathing have a much greater significance. The most important goal in both traditions is to put an end to avidya, false knowledge.

THE SCRIPTURES OF VEDA

Veda means knowledge and the scriptures are divided into four parts (samitha):

1. The Rigveda (roughly the 30th century BC) is the oldest part of the Vedic scriptures, where yoga and the Saraswati river are mentioned.

These Vedas are hymns that are recited and serve as regulations for various ritu-als. To perform the rituals successfully, various yoga techniques were developed to strengthen the ability to concentrate.

2. The Samaveda are Vedas with sung hymns.

3. The Yajurveda are Vedas with ritual texts.

4. The Atharvaveda are Vedas with magic formulas.

According to the Vedic worldview, our world is a reflection of the cosmic world. By maintaining the cosmic order in our world, one can create a harmonious existence. To get an inner picture of the cosmic order, followers use various yoga techniques such as regulated breathing, mantra singing and concentration exercises.

These samithas are the first part of the wood. Three more texts are included:

1. Brahmana: comments on the videos that explain the rituals of each samitha.

2. Aranyaka: "Forest books".

3. The Upanishads: The last part of the Vedas and often seen as the most important. This esoteric text describes the worldview found in Vedanta and is the most famous philosophical system in India.

The Upanishads are based on four basic concepts:

1. That the brahman (world soul) is identical to the atman (the human soul), which means that the creative energy of the universe is identical to our inner self.

2. The realization that the unity of everything leads to spiritual enlightenment – moksha. This insight frees us from the cycle of rebirth.

3. The law of karma, which means that our thoughts and actions affect our future.

4. If you do not reach insight, you are born according to your karma.

In the Katha, Svetasvarata and Maitri Upanishads, you can find descriptions of yoga exercises as well as Samkhya concepts and performances, which indicates that yoga has been associated with Samkhya from an early age.

"IT IS THE HIGHEST STATE: WHEN THE FIVE SENSE
ORGANS AND THE MIND HAVE CALMED DOWN AND THE IN-
TELLECT IS IMMOBILE. THIS CONTROL OF THE SENSES THEY
CALL YOGA. THEN HE IS FREE FROM DISTURBANCES, FOR
YOGA IS BOTH ORIGIN AND CESSATION."

(KATHA-UPANISHAD 6.10-11)

"BY HOLDING THE BODY WITH ITS TOP THREE PARTS RIGHT
AND GETTING THE FEELINGS AND SENSES TO GO IN THE
HEART, THE SAGE CROSSES ALL DANGEROUS RIVERS WITH
BRAHMAN AS A BOAT.

WHILE CONTROLLING BREATHING AND ALL
MOVEMENTS, HE SHOULD BREATHE THROUGH HIS NOSE,
WITH CONTROLLED BREATHING SOUNDS THE WISE CON-
TROL HIS MIND AS HE STEERS A CHARIOT DRAWN BY WILD
HORSES.

IN AN EVEN AND CLEAN PLACE, FREE FROM PEBBLES, FIRE
AND SAND, NEAR RUNNING WATER, IN ONE PLACE THE MIND
FINDS ATTRACTIVE AND TO WHICH THE EYE DOES NOT
REACT AS UGLY, IN A HIDDEN
PLACE SHELTERED FROM THE WIND, HE SHOULD PRACTICE
YOGA."

(SVETASVATARA-UPANISHAD 2.8-2.10)

THE MAHABHARATA

*Yoga is also mentioned in the Mahabharata, which belongs to the category of iti-
hasa (history) and which is one of two great epic works in Hinduism, especially
in Books 12 and 13 where yoga is described in close connection with Samkhya:*

"WHAT YOGIS SEE IS THE SAME AS
THE FOLLOWERS OF SAMKHYA PERCEIVE. HE IS A SAGE WHO
SEES SAMKHYA AND YOGA AS THE SAME."

(MAHABHARATA 12.293.30)

*The Bhagavad Gita is a mythological work of poetry and the most important
scripture in Bhakti yoga. This great epic belongs to the Mahabharata and was
added about 700 AD. It is seen as a summary of the Upanishads. Here, Krishna
is described as the master of yoga, and yoga is seen as a disciplined method of
achieving a goal. Three yoga paths are described – Jnana, Karma and Bhakti, of
which Bhakti is seen as the highest.*

"IT IS BETTER TO FOLLOW ONE'S DHARMA BADLY THAN
ANOTHER'S FLAWLESS."

(BHAGAVAD GITA 3.35)

"WHILE SITTING THERE, HE SHOULD PRACTICE YOGA TO
CLEAR THE MIND, KEEP THE MIND ATTACHED TO AN OBJECT
AND RESTRAIN THE MIND AND
EMOTIONS."

(BHAGAVAD GITA 6.12)

DIFFERENT YOGA PATHS

As said, yoga is a broad tradition with many branches and techniques. Down the ages, masters have developed various techniques for spiritual enlightenment. There are no direct boundaries between the yoga paths, but everyone goes in some way into each. Within a yoga tradition, one can use many different techniques.

KARMA YOGA – THE WAY OF ACTION

Karma yoga is a way of action and is mainly suitable for people who are outgoing. It means working, performing social activities and helping other people with no thought of getting anything in return. Karma yoga is a continuation of the Vedic sacrificial doctrine where sacrifices were made to the gods. In the Bhagavad Gita, sacrificial acts mean one is loyal to the doctrine of warning, that they follow their dharma and the class they belong to.

Today, Karma yoga is more about selfless, moral action. The job itself is not the most important, but rather one's attitude during its execution. One's attitude determines whether the action or job is perceived as liberating or binding, painful and hard. Whatever you choose to do, make sure you always do your best. If you can do the job better, you make sure to do it. One should not let negative thoughts hold one back, such as fear of criticism. You should also not feel bound by or dependent on your job, but be prepared to leave it if necessary. Mahatma Gandhi and Mother Teresa are two famous karma yogis.

BHAKTI YOGA – THE WAY OF DEDICATION

This path is suitable for people who are emotional with nature. One surrenders oneself to God through prayers, worship and rituals, driven by the power of love and experiencing God as love itself. Being devoted and loving towards a personal god is considered to lead to salvation. Chanting and singing God's name is a central part of bhakti yoga.

RAJA YOGA – THE WAY OF MEDITATION

Often called the royal way, Raja yoga involves the control of thoughts. One trains the mind through meditation and transforms mental and physical energy into spiritual energy. Raja yoga is also called Ashtanga yoga, which refers to "eight-step yoga", which should systematically lead to control of the mind. When the body and energy are under control and in harmony, meditation takes place by itself.

Ashtanga yoga's eight steps – the Yoga Sutras of Patanjali:

1. Yamas – five basic ideas about moral discipline, "do not do":

Ahimsa – do not use violence.
Sathyam – be true.
Brahmacharya – moderation, control over desire, chastity.
Asteya – do not steal.
Aparighara – do not be greedy.

2. Niyamas – five basic ideas about ethical action, "should do":

Saucha – external and internal cleanliness, such as thoughts, speech, and hygiene.
Santosha – contentment.
Tapas – restraint, self-discipline.
Swadhyaya – studies.
Ishvara pranidhana – the worship of God.

3. Asana – body position.
The lotus position. To be able to sit completely immobile so as not to be distracted by the physical body during meditation.

4. Pranayamas – controlled breathing.
Controlled breathing to control the prana in the body, which calms the mind.

5. Pratyahara – directs the sense organs inward.
Calms the mind when you are not disturbed by the environment and external stimuli.

6. Dharana – concentration.
Concentration is achieved by focusing on an object.

7. Dhyana – meditation.
After a long period of concentration, meditation is achieved.

8. Samadhi – ecstasy.
Prolonged meditation leads to ecstasy. The yogi becomes at one with the object of meditation when the movements of the mind cease.

JNANA YOGA – THE WAY OF KNOWLEDGE

This is perhaps the most difficult path because it requires a strong will and a sharp intellect. It is mainly suitable for theoretically inclined people. A Jnana yogi comes to an understanding of the transient and the eternal in life by studying Vedanta, which belongs to the Upanishads, the last part of the Vedic scriptures. It is difficult to reach spiritual insight through theoretical knowledge; therefore, it is important to practice other yoga paths as a preparation. Ramana Maharishi is a well-known jnana yogi.

THE MANTRA

The mantra consists of words and syllables that carry a special vibration and affect the mind and body in a positive and strengthening way. According to tradition, mantras have been used to reach a deeper plane of consciousness.

With mantra meditation, you calm your thoughts and mind. By repeating the same mantra over and over again, you do not give the mind any new stimulus, instead allowing the subconscious mind to wake up. Old thoughts and memories have an opportunity to come to the surface and the subconscious mind can be purified from them. One looks more clearly at life and is no longer governed by old thought patterns. In the same way that asanas are meant to strengthen and purify the body, the mantra is meant to calm and "clean up" the mind.

In yoga, it is believed that everything in the universe consists of energy that vibrates differently. Mantras consist of a high vibration that should have a beneficial and positive effect on our body. When we recite or sing a mantra, we begin to vibrate at the same rate. In our palate we have eighty-four meridian points that affect the pituitary gland, the pineal gland and the chemical balance of the brain. When we pronounce certain mantras, the tongue hits these meridian points, which can increase mental clarity and awareness.

Most often one recites a mantra one hundred and eight times. Our physical and subtle body has seventy-two thousand energy channels called nadis. One hundred and eight of these meet at hrit padma, the area around the Anahata chakra. By repeating a mantra one hundred and eight times, the whole physical and subtle body is permeated by its energy.

THE GAYATRI MANTRA

The Gayatri mantra is said to be the oldest mantra, with its origins in the Rig-veda Vedic scripture. It is sometimes called Savitri because in the mantra one prays to Deva Savitr, the sun god who was worshipped during the Vedic period (the sun before sunrise is called Savitri and after sunrise surya). The Gayatri mantra is also found in other Hindu texts such as the Bhagavad Gita, and is of great importance in Hindu traditions. It is taught to children when they turn eight years old.

The Gayatri mantra is said to heal physically, mentally and emotionally. It expands consciousness, promotes spiritual development and develops one's intellectual potential, knowledge and wisdom. It acts sattvic.

THE GAYATRI MANTRA

Om bhur bhuvaha svaha
Tat savitur varenyam
Bhargo devasya dhimahi
Dhiyo yonah prachodayat

"Praise to the source of all things. It is due to you that we attain true happiness on the planes of earth, astral, casual. It is due to your transcendent nature that you are worthy of being worshiped and adored. Ignite us with your all-pervading light"

MAHAMRITYUNJAYA

This mantra also has its roots in the Rigveda Vedic literature and is also called the tryambakam mantra. It is dedicated to "the three-eyed": an epithet of Rudra, who later came to be characterized as Shiva.

The mahamrityunjaya mantra provides peace and protection. It is said to heal physically, mentally and emotionally. It counteracts rajas.

THE MAHAMRITYUNJAYA MANTRA

Om triambakam yajamahe
Sugandhim pushti vardanam
Urvarukamiva bandhanan
Mrityor muksheeya mamritat

"SHELTER ME, THE THREE-EYED LORD SHIVA.
BLESS ME WITH HEALTH AND IMMORTALITY
AND SEVER ME FROM THE CLUTCHES OF DEATH,
EVEN AS A CUCUMBER IS CUT FROM ITS CREEPER"

THE INFLUENCE OF TANTRISM ON YOGA

During the post-classical period, it was primarily tantrism that came to influence the yoga tradition. According to tantrism, the divine power (Kundalini Shakti) in the human body is inactive. This brings the physical body into focus for ritual exercises, a new phenomenon in the spiritual history of India.

THE BHAGAVAD GITA

The Bhagavad Gita (the "Song of God") is the god Krishna's song. It is a mythological work in Sanskrit, and an independent story in the great epic, the Mahabharata. In the Bhagavad Gita, a dialogue takes place between Krishna and Prince Arjuna, just before the great battle of Kurukshetra. Arjuna faces a dilemma: his duty as a warrior is to follow his dharma and begin the battle, but at the same time he sees it as a terrible sin to kill the many great men, relatives and gurus who are in the opponents' army. To accompany the prince through this difficult decision, Krishna teaches him various forms of yoga. The story takes place about five thousand years ago.

The Bhagavad Gita can be seen as a summary of the Upanishads. Each chapter ends with the Bhagavad Gita being called Upanishad. Krishna says in Bhagavad Gita 3.3 that there have been two paths since ancient times:

1.) Karma yoga – the way of action, that is to do one's duty without worrying about the outcome.
2.) Jnana yoga – the way of knowledge, that is knowledge of the self (atman).

Other ways are variants of these.

Krishna shows his vishvarupa, his universal form, for Arjuna on the battlefield at Kurukshetra. The Bhagavad Gita consists of eighteen chapters:

1. Arjuna lets Krishna pull his chariot to a place in the middle of the two armies. When Arjuna sees his relatives on the opposite side of Kurus, he loses his motivation and decides not to fight.

2. Krishna explains to Arjuna that his concern about fighting against his relatives and gurus is unjustified because only the body can be killed, while the eternal self is immortal. Krishna reminds Arjuna that as a warrior he must follow, his dharma, and wage war.

3. Arjuna asks why he has to fight if knowledge is more important than action. Krishna emphasizes that the right way to act is to carry out one's duties for good, but without clinging to the results.

4. Krishna says that he has lived through many births and always taught yoga to protect the righteous and to annihilate the unrighteous. He emphasizes the importance of trusting a guru.

5. Arjuna asks Krishna if it is better to refrain from action or to perform actions. Krishna replies that both ways can be good, but that action, karma yoga, is the highest.

6. Krishna describes the correct position of meditation and the process of achieving samadhi.

7. Krishna teaches the way of knowledge, Jnana yoga.

8. Krishna defines the terms brahman, adhyatma, karma, atman, adhibhuta and adhidaiva, and explains how to remember him at the moment of death and attain a higher state.

9. Krishna describes panentheism, "all beings are in me", as a way of remembering him in all circumstances.

10. Krishna declares that he is the ultimate source of all material and spiritual worlds. Arjuna recognizes Krishna as the supreme being and quotes famous scholars who have done the same.

11. At Arjuna's request, Krishna demonstrates a theophany, its "universal form", Visvarupa: a terrifying creature that is turned in all directions at the same time, which spreads the radiation from a thousand suns around it, and which contains all other beings and all matter that exists.

12. Krishna describes the process of devotion, Bhakti yoga.

13. Krishna describes matter (Prakriti) and consciousness (Purusha).

14. Krishna talks about the three states, gunas, which together constitute all beings.

15. Krishna describes a symbolic tree, which represents the material existence, its roots in heaven and its foliage on earth. He explains that this tree should be felled with the "axe of indifference" so that one can move on to a higher state.

16. Krishna describes the human traits of divine and demonic beings. He advises that the higher state can be achieved by renouncing lust, anger and greed and by distinguishing right actions from wrong deeds through buddhi and advice from scriptures and thereby acting right.

17. Krishna talks about the three variants of faith, knowledge, actions, and even of eating habits, which are linked to the three gunas.

18. In conclusion, Krishna asks Arjuna to abandon all dharma and solely submit to him. He describes this as the ultimate and final perfection of life.

LESSON NO. 5

LONG SHAVASANA – DEAD MAN'S POSTURE/RELAXATION.

SUPTA PAWANMUKTASANA – THE LEG LOCK.

SHAVASANA – DEAD MAN'S POSTURE.

SURYA NAMASKARA – SUN SALUTATION WITHOUT BREATHING.

SHAVASANA – DEAD MAN'S POSTURE.

PASCHIMOTTANASANA – THE PLIERS.

MATSYASANA – THE FISH.

SHAVASANA – DEAD MAN'S POSTURE.

SHAVA UDARAKARSHANASANA – THE UNIVERSAL POSITION.

SHAVASANA – DEAD MAN'S POSTURE.

SARPASANA – THE SNAKE

SHASHANKASANA – THE HARE.

SHAVASANA – DEAD MAN'S POSTURE.

YOGA NIDRA – DEEP RELAXATION.

KAYA STHAIRYAM & AJAPA JAPA – STEP 1 + 2 – MEDITATION.

END WITH – HARI OM TAT SAT, 3 TIMES

THEN – OM SRI DURGAYAI NAMAH, 1 TIME.

INSTRUCTIONS FOR ASANAS LESSON NO. 5

LONG SHAVASANA – DEAD MAN'S POSTURE/RELAXATION.

Execution: See module 1.

SUPTA PAWANMUKTASANA – THE LEG LOCK.

Execution: See module no. 1 & 2.

SHAVASANA – DEAD MAN'S POSTURE.

Execution: See module no. 1 & 2.

SURYA NAMASKARA – SUN SALUTATION WITHOUT BREATHING.

Execution: See module 3.

SHAVASANA – DEAD MAN'S POSTURE.

Execution: See module no. 1 & 2.

PASCHIMOTTANASANA – THE PLIERS.

Execution: See module 2.

MATSYASANA – THE FISH.

Execution: See module 2.

SHAVASANA – DEAD MAN'S POSTURE.

Execution: See module no. 1 & 2.

SHAVA UDARAKARSHANASANA – THE UNIVERSAL POSITION.

Execution: See module 1 & 2.

SHAVASANA – DEAD MAN'S POSTURE.

Execution: See module no. 1 & 2.

BHUJANGASANA – THE COBRA.

Execution: See module 2.

SHASHANKASANA – THE HARE.

Execution: See module 1 & 2.

SHAVASANA – DEAD MAN'S POSTURE.

Execution: See module no. 1 & 2.

YOGA NIDRA – DEEP RELAXATION.

Execution: See module 3.

KAYA STHAIRYAM & AJAPA JAPA – STEP 1 + 2 – MEDITATION.

Execution: See module 3.

ANAHATA CHAKRA (READ ABOUT THE CHAKRANA IN MODUL 4)

To practice regularly for a month.

Chakra and kshetram localization/activation & purification with Ram chanting. Press one finger against the heart and one finger at the corresponding point at the spine. Inhale and hold your breath as you experience the pulsation from the chakra and visualize the color while saying Yam silently to yourself. You can also visualize the yantra. Exhale and then continue in the same way for 5-10 minutes.

Anahata chakra bhedan i matsyasana. Practice matsyasana (the fish), then inhale through the heart and pierce the spine and chakras. Feel how the whole astral body expands like a hot air balloon and you experience the chakra attri-butes. You feel light – lighter than air, you float high up in the clouds, experience the blue sky, and experience boundless love and happiness throughout your body. Boundless happiness in every little cell of the body. When you exhale – you exhale through the spine and heart and the body contracts slightly. Continue for 2-5 minutes.

KNOWLEDGE TEST MODULE 5

ANSWER AS FULLY AS YOU CAN, THEN CHECK IF YOU ANSWERED CORRECTLY. PRACTICE UNTIL YOU KNOW THE ANSWERS BY HEART.

1. WHAT IS HINDUISM?

2. DESCRIBE THE TRADITIONS OF HINDUISM.

3. DESCRIBE THE SCRIPTURES.

4. DESCRIBE THE IMPORTANCE OF YOGA IN HINDUISM.

5. DESCRIBE MANTRAS.

6. EXPLAIN AND RECEIVE GAYATRI MANTRA.

7. EXPLAIN AND RECEIVE THE MAHAMRITYUNJAYA MANTRA.

8. WHAT IS BHAGAVAD GITA?

9. TALK ABOUT ANAHATA CHAKRA, ITS ELEMENT, YANTRA, CO-LOR, NUMBER OF PETALS AND ATTRIBUTES.

10. DESCRIBE SOME POWERFUL EXERCISES TO ACTIVATE, CLEAN AND BALANCE ANAHATA CHAKRA.

MODULE 6

TANTRA & TATTWA SHUDDHI. WE ARE STUDYING PANCHA TATTWA – THE FIVE ELEMENTS

We study tantra and the ancient technique of purifying the five elements – tattwa shuddhi. We study the Vishuddhi chakra and practice our exercises to cleanse, balance and activate the chakra. We continue to practice in the role of yoga teacher with lesson no. 6 of 8.

Knowledge test: Answer the questions related to module 6. Practice lesson no. 6 with at least 1 participant and humbly accept feedback from them. Ask questions afterward – how was the pace, did you keep to time, did you speak loudly enough, and how well did you understand the exercises?

TANTRA YOGA

TANTRA, MANTRA & YANTRA

The word tantra refers to those religious literary works in which mysticism and magic play the main role and form the group of ritual books belonging to the mysticism of later Hinduism.

Tantra books are intended to be a guide in the use of magical and mysterious formulas and are often in the form of dialogues between Shiva and Durga. The word tantra comes from Sanskrit and is a combination of the words; tanoti and trayati, which can be translated as expansion and liberation. Tantra as a method is about expanding the mind and releasing the dormant potential energy that exists in man. Tantra sadhana – different tantric rituals – all evoke Kundalini Shakti in different ways.

To expand the mind, we must learn not to be controlled by our sensory experiences. When we are controlled by our senses and our ego, we categorize all our experiences into what we "like" and "do not like", which are called raga and dwesha. This categorization leads to suffering and inhibits our development and our ability to see pure, true knowledge. As we develop and expand the mind, we gradually develop our intuitive ability which is said to be the source of true, eternal, and right knowledge.

In our daily lives, we perceive and take in our surroundings through our senses. If we instead learn to see, feel, listen and turn the mind inwards, we can create an inner experience about ourselves and thus expand the mind. By releasing the energy (Shakti) and merging it with consciousness (Shiva), we create a homogeneous consciousness and experience Kundalini, which is the very purpose of tantra. The difference between tantra and most other spiritual philosophical paths is that in tantra you do not set up a lot of rules that you have to live by.

Everyone has an opportunity to develop, regardless of where they are in their development. One can be sensualist or spiritualist, atheist or theist, poor or rich, strong or weak; the road is for everyone to discover. There are a total of sixty-four different tantras and each one describes a different approach to mind control and expansion. Tantric techniques are often mistaken for being dirty and bizarre when alcohol, drugs and sex are included in certain exercises and rituals. However, it is not used as a means of pleasure but as a means of expanding the mind.

Tantra describes Shakti, the subtle form of energy as a coiled snake at the bottom of the body at the end of the spine, at the Mooladhara chakra. Shiva, the pure consciousness is said to have its seat on top of the head in the Sahasrara chakra. To awaken the Kundalini energy, which in most people is dormant, one must first increase the flow and amount of prana, the vital energy down to the Mooladhara chakra. Then Kundalini Shakti can be directed up to the Sahasrara chakra. On its way up along the spine, Kundalini Shakti passes six chakras or energy pools. When Kundalini Shakti rises, they are charged with energy. The chakras act as nodes for our nadis energy channels, and these vibrate at different intensities. Chakras carry dormant creative forces that are partially evident in our daily lives and whose full potential can only emerge when kundalini Shakti have passed through them on their way up to Shiva.

Tantric exercises are divided into three steps in the form of upasana or worship:

Shuddhi – purification of the gross, subtle and psychic elements or tattwas.
Sthiti – enlightenment by concentration achieved by purifying the elements.
Arpana – insight into the cosmic consciousness.

Tantric exercises can be easily distinguished from other non-tantric exercises by the sacred formulas, symbols and rituals used. Through worship and rituals, we want to attract higher subtle forces as well as our inner forces. Tattwa shuddhi belongs to one of the tantric rituals.

FIRST STEP – CLEANING THE ELEMENT

One of the first introductory tantric rituals is tattwa shuddhi, also known as bhuta shuddhi,which aims to purify our elements.

In tantra, tattwa/bhuta shuddhi is used to transform the pranic flow from our elements so it returns to the original unmanifested form – Shakti. As long as the prana flows in our external organs and is fixed in our elements, our consciousness will be limited to the external world. The energy/consciousness is thus fixed and limited to our physical body through our elements. By releasing it, we can also make it expand.

The first step towards expansion is a purification of our basic physical, mental, psychic and pranic structures. In yoga, there are various purifying techniques aimed at this: prana shuddhi, nadi shuddhi, vak shuddhi, manas shuddhi, etc. But the practice of tattwa/bhuta shuddhi, according to the ancient tantras, is comprehensive. The techniques used in tattwa shuddhi are:

Nyasa – concentration on the body.

Prana prathishta – placement of life and prana in mandala.

Panchopchara – five things sacrificed in the worship of tattwan.

Japa – mantra repetition.

In many of the ancient tantric texts, tattwa shuddhi is described as an important technique to move development forward and gain greater insight. Tattwa shuddhi strengthens our personal experiences of energy and pure consciousness. It is not enough to "know" intellectually that all matter has its origin in the pure consciousness, it must be experienced. Personal experience is the core of tantra and can be made possible with the help of tattwa shuddhi.

By focusing on tattwa yantras, we not only increase the prana in the body but also affect each chakra. Each tattwa is tied to a chakra. Charging each chakra prepares the awakening of the Kundalini Shakti and facilitates its path up to the Sahasrara chakra. Tattwa shuddhi also develops our ability to concentrate (dharana), which leads to spontaneous meditation (dhyana), which in turn leads to awareness of the subtle essence behind matter and form (tattwa jnana).

BRIEF DESCRIPTION OF TATTWA SHUDDHI

With the help of meditation and self-reflection, the elements that make up the mind and body are purified and transformed. Tattwa shuddhi is a dynamic form of meditation and self-reflection. It is not a passive form where you have to focus on the same symbol for a long time. During the implementation of tattwa shuddhi, one easily deepens the mind, by creating images of tattwa yantras (geometric images of the elements), papa purusha (the sinful man) and the mandala of prana shakti (the form of the creative energy).

You start the exercise by creating a mental image of the elements and their respective yantra in the body. You witness how the elements are born from each other and you thus sink deeper into yourself. When one discovers the universal cosmic energy within, one uses the power to heal inner imbalances. With the help of a higher state of consciousness and a stronger mind, it is easier to heal imbalances. After this, an inner image of the elements is again created, but in reverse order. Towards the end, one visualizes an image of prana shakti, the energy that is manifested through the elements. Finally, apply bhasma or ash to the body.

Tattwa shuddhi can be used as an aid to entering a meditative state or as a complete sadhana in itself.

To get the most out of the exercise, you should have practiced Hatha yoga and ajapa japa for a long time. The mind and body must be in good condition. You must be able to sit still for a long time without the mind being disturbed by the surroundings. Just before the exercise, it is an important preparation to turn the mind inward which is best done with the help of pranayamas and trataka. You should also have a good knowledge of the location of the chakras in the body and how the prana moves along the sushumna. If you are ill, you should wait until you have recovered before you start practicing tattwa shuddhi.

CLEANING PROCESS

Tattwa shuddhi is a process that cleanses the elements of our body and purifies the senses connected to those elements. The sense of hearing is purified using mantra repetition; the sight by observing yantras and mandalas; the feeling and our tactile nerves by applying bhasma or ash to the body; the sense of smell by breathing exercises; and the sense of taste by eating sattvic food or by fasting.

Tattwa shuddhi does not only cleanse our physical body but cleanses the layers of all of our bodies. In addition to our physical body, we have several other bodies relating to the invisible parts of the mind that are affected by samskaras (latent impressions) which create sankalpa and vikalpa (thoughts/counter-thoughts) in our conscious mind.

Imbalances in the various bodies manifest themselves in the form of anxiety, distress, depression, and fear. We often find it difficult to cure these conditions in the same way as physical illnesses. In the long run, these imbalances affect our life and our personality. Our body is an extension of our mind and each affects the other. Since the mind largely controls our body and its functions, it is as important to purify your mental mind as it is your physical body.

In tantra, it is said that there is no action or thought that is unclean or wrong in itself. The unclean lies in wrong perception and judgment. Through the sadhana, we can come to an understanding of this and thus fight it. Without purifying the subtle levels of the mind, it is impossible to reach higher levels of consciousness. An unclean mind cannot focus or concentrate. By harmonizing the flow of prana in the body, separating the intellect and ego from the consciousness, one can purify the different levels of the mind so that one becomes the experiencer and the witness at the same time.

CLEANING OF THE ELEMENT

Tattwa shuddhi is a unique technique because it purifies the whole person from the coarsest layers to the most subtle. The first step in the cleansing process is to wash and cleanse the physical body; apply bhasma or ash; and fast and control food intake. Tantra emphasizes the importance of doing all everyday chores with awareness and presence. Everything you do, how you sit, walk, talk, wash, etc. reflects your state of mind. Tattwa shuddhi is thus a purification process that covers all twenty-four hours of the day. However, the first step in the process of physical purity is more about discipline than raising awareness.

The second step in the process purifies the subtle levels. You use your mind and prana. Internal forces are aroused and controlled by the elements. By refining the elements, the energy increases so that they can vibrate harmoniously which creates a balance that leads to an increased inner awareness. By repeating the bija mantra and visualizing the yantra of each tattwa, one can dissolve deeply rooted samskaras and archetypes that prevent us from experiencing infinite consciousness.

PRANA SHAKTI

In our body, the prana moves in a specific pattern, which means that vibrations are created at different frequency levels. The vibrational frequencies build up our physical body as well as our subtle organs. We can see and feel the physical organs and their constituents while the subtle organs are experienced. In tantra and yoga, these subtle organs are called chakras, nadis, Kundalini Shakti, chitta Shakti, prana vayu and pancha tattwa.

The prana exists in the microcosm and macrocosm. Without it, we would not function or exist. We would not have the ability to see, hear or move. Most of us have too little flow of prana in our body which leads to fatigue and exhaustion.

The cosmic prana in our body is represented by Kundalini Shakti, which has its seat in the Mooladhara chakra. When its full potential is awakened, it rises along the central nervous system of our physical body which in our pranic body is called the sushumna nadi. Kundalini Shakti also manifests itself in our larger six chakras.

Each chakra consists of one element. In Mooladhara there are elements of the earth – prithvi tattwa; in Swadhisthana elements of water – apas tattwa; in Manipura elements of fire – agni tattwa; in Anahata elements of air – vayu tattwa; and in Vishuddhi elements of ether or space – akasha tattwa. The element that controls the chakra reveals the frequency at which the chakra vibrates. Our entire consciousness, thoughts and actions are controlled by the degree of activity of the chakra. Pingala nadi supplies chakras with energy and Kundalini Shakti activates and opens them up to their full potential. When our chakras are only partially activated, we become limited in our way of acting and experiencing. In tattwa shuddhi, we affect each chakra directly by concentrating on each tattwa.

MANDALA BY PRANA SHAKTI

In tantra, there is a tradition of symbolizing the various aspects of man in the form of mandalas. Mandalas represent the human subconscious and unconscious mind. By concentrating on these images, we can relax samskaras or archetypes that stand in the way of our creativity and knowledge. In tattwa shuddhi sadhana, an image of prana Shakti is created in the form of a beautiful goddess who has a powerful effect on us.

Prana Shakti as a goddess is red. Red is a base color that stands for raja guna. The color also symbolizes the dynamic quality of prana. Her six arms symbolize the efficiency she has in everything she undertakes. In each hand, she holds a tool that symbolizes different aspects of human existence. Her three eyes stand for clairvoyance and the lotus flower on which she sits for the development of powers and siddhis

ANTAH KARANA

Antah karana is man's inner tool and consists of four parts: buddhi (intellect), ahamkara (ego), manas (thoughts and counter-thoughts) and chitta (memory). According to tantra and yoga, these four are the core of which consciousness acts from the outside. Antah karana is unique and can only be found in humans. In lower life forms (animals and plant species) antah karana exists only in a precursor. Plants and animals act instinctively and not based on ego, intellect or thoughts. Antah karana is what sets man apart from other species.

Through antah karana, the human consciousness interprets, classifies and perceives everything that concerns the past, present and future. It can be said that it is a recipient who receives and sends out impressions. In antah karana, in addition to the knowledge of this life and what happens here, there is also the knowledge of the entire universe and cosmos. This knowledge is often unmanifested and dormant in humans. It is part of human evolution to refine the frequency of antah karana.

Antah karana is an instrument that we have built up through all our incarnations. It carries all the impressions of our past lives. Antah karana determines the individual's future actions based on previous experiences and knowledge. These experiences and knowledge are often unconscious to us unless we develop our inner vision and experience of the cosmos. Through tantric techniques, we can learn to see and control antah karana which is part of our evolution.

DIMENSIONS OF THE MIND

In yoga, the mind is divided into four parts: jagriti (conscious mind), swapana (unconscious mind), sushpati (subconscious mind) and turya (our transcendental mind). In modern psychology, only the first three are mentioned.

Antah karana acts based on the conscious, subconscious and unconscious mind. Manas and chitta, which are part of the conscious and subconscious mind, control thoughts and actions on the conscious and subconscious plane. Buddhi and ahamkara constantly exist to varying degrees in the conscious, subconscious and unconscious mind. Since all of these have arisen from the same principle, which is Shakti, they influence each other intensively.

The three gunas, sattva, rajas and tamas lay the foundation for antah karana. These three cosmic principles have a great influence on manas, chitta and buddhi and thus affect our experiences. The fourth sense, turya is not affected by the interplay between the three gunas. Turya can only be developed by refining antah karana through sadhana. In tattwa shuddhi we learn to perceive antah karana and use its full potential for further spiritual development.

BUDDHI

Buddhi is the principle that most closely resembles pure consciousness. It motivates us to follow our dharma. Sattvic buddhi is characterized by wisdom, happiness, perseverance, calm, self-control and discernment. Under the influence of rajas, some defects occur, which means that the ability to distinguish deteriorates and even actions are affected by wrong knowledge and avidya. A tamasic buddhi acts under the ego is judgmental and permeated by misinterpretations of the outside world. In tattwa shuddhi, the principle of buddhi is meditated on sattvic. This removes the qualities of rajas and tamas that stand in the way of sattvic buddhi.

AHAMKARA

Aham means "I" and ahamkara is the ego or what one experiences as the "self". The ego is the core of individualism, which makes us identify with matter. Ahamkara is very subtle. At the same time as the ego binds man to objective experiences, it is the core that must be opened to experience unity. Without the ego, man would not be aware of his existence. On the conscious plane, the ego acts through our physical body, senses and mind. On the subconscious plane, it acts through our astral body and dreams. During deep sleep, the ego withdraws while during meditation it functions as the inner consciousness.
Sattvic ahamkara acts as a catalyst for self-realization. Ahamkara usually takes up the comrades' and underlying experiences from the subconscious mind, but

in a sattvic state, this stops. Rajasic ahamkara raises the identification with the "self" and leads to restlessness and a constant need to do something. A tamasic ahamkara strengthens painful and negative samskaras which causes fear and doubt. Through tattwa shuddhi we can learn to see how the ego works and thus stop identifying with it.

MANAS AND CHITTA

Manas and chitta represent the external mind: thoughts that come up in our waking state as well as during dreams. Chitta is the core of all experiences in the form of samskaras, archetypes and memories. Manas, i.e. our thoughts, are chitta's tools that coexist, and by which archetypes and memories are expressed. Manas and chitta do not work individually but are influenced by both buddhi and ahamkara. In a sattvic state, our manas are steady, focused and concentrated. Under the influence of rajas our senses are activated which creates an imbalance in our intellect. Tamasic manas makes the intellect and the senses sluggish and inactive.

When chitta is in a sattvic state, our senses are withdrawn so that consciousness remains undisturbed. Under the influence of rajas, rajasic awakened samskaras in chitta in the form of vikalpa (fantasy) and viparayaya (wrong knowledge). In that state, chitta contains both types of cohabitation, knowledge and ignorance, passion and freedom. When tamas prevail in chitta, unwanted samskaras will come up in the form of vasanas (deep-rooted desires).

The coexistence of a negative nature can only be eliminated through reflection, dharana and dhyana. Tattwa shuddhi helps us to enter into meditation which has the purpose of liberating the consciousness. Only then can we reflect on the structure of the elements and influence them.

PANCHA TATTWA – THE FIVE ELEMENTS

All matter is made up of five elements, akasha, vayu, agni, apas and prithvi. The elements lay the foundation for the creation and make it last. The elements affect every aspect of our life, thoughts and actions. In yoga, it is important to learn how these elements work to be able to control and influence them and our lives. In tantric texts, the science behind the elements is described.

The elements form a kind of chain where they are born from each other. Akasha is the first element of the process. Akasha consists of subtle matter and energy, which rests in consciousness. When the energy in akasha begins to vibrate, movement is created, vayu tattwa starts to take shape. Vayu stands for the movement that permeates everything. The intense movement creates heat, which causes the next element in the joint (agni) to be created. Agni tattwa has a slower vibration than vayu. This allows the heat to cool down and form apas, the elements of water. The vibration and movement of the apas are minimal. The last element, prithvi, occurs when the movement/vibration is further reduced. Apas solidify and become the elements of the earth. The elements should be seen as an extension of pure consciousness, not as separate existing parts.

During evolution, tattwas have been further developed through tanmatras. Tanmatra is the quality through which tattwas are perceived. Akasha is perceived through shaba tanmatra (sound), vayu through sparsha tanmatra (feeling), agni through roopa tanmatra (vision), apas through rasa tanmatra (taste) and prithvi through gandha tanmatra (smell). When we are born, we are created from the roughest form of the elements. In tattwa shuddhi we create an experience of the elements in their subtle form to develop spiritually.

The Patanjali Yoga Sutras state that each element consists of five different characters. To take control of the elements one must practice samyama which is a combination of concentration, meditation and samadhi. Patanjali called this bhuta jaya, "knowledge of the elements". The first character of the five elements is the rough form that relates to experiences that we take in through our senses: sound, touch, form, taste and smell. The second character relates to the quality of the elements: the liquid property of water, the heat of fire, the movement of air and the space of ether. The third character is the subtle form of tanmatras. Here,

*tattwas are experienced in the form of subtle sounds, sensations, form, smell
and taste and are often called mental visions. The fourth aspect of the elements
relates to the three gunas (sattva, rajas and tamas) which are an essential part of
the elements. One should strive to transform the qualities of rajasic and tamasic
into more sattvic to develop spiritually. Tattwa shuddhi enables this change. The
fifth aspect of the elements is called arthavattwa which stands for the actual goal
of the elements. The scriptures describe that it is for the liberation and enjoyment
of consciousness from matter that the elements have developed.*

*The elements are characterized by shaba (sound) and warn (color) and are
created by the vibration in the element. The color refers to the energy frequency
of the element. Akasha is black as the vibration is minimal. Vayu vibrates in the
frequency of blue, agni in red, apas in white and prithvi in yellow. The second
manifestation of the energy of the elements is sound in the form of bija mantras.
Bija mantra for akasha is Ham, for vayu – Yam, agni – Ram, apas – Vam and
for prithvi – Lam.*

*Sound and color together build the form of energy. Akasha is experienced as
a circle, vayu as a hexagon, agni as an inverted triangle, apas as a horizontal
crescent moon and prithvi as a yellow square.*

AKASHA TATTWA *– the element of space.*
*Akasha can be described as the space or emptiness between two objects or
matter. Akasha is the most subtle of all the elements and is almost motionless. It
stands for the whole spectrum of sounds, from the rough to the subtle and acts
as a carrier for the sound. The vibration of the element is so subtle that it cannot
be experienced with external senses. It is said that ether moves at a higher
speed than sound. Akasha tattwa is boundless and permeates the entire cosmos,
therefore it has the shape of a circle. It is not of matter as we know it and cannot
be experienced physically. Tattwa jnanis has discovered akasha by refining the
rough mind. Because of this quality, tantra has described the element as mental
(not physical) and as the "space of the mind" behind closed eyes, which is called*

chidakasha. Tattwa akasha stands for the space in the body between our organs. On a mental level, tattwa akasha controls the emotions and passions of man. The best time for meditation and concentration is when akasha flows in the body, which happens about five minutes every hour. The element has its seat on top of the head. Mentally it relates to our unconscious mind and its psychic centers are the Vishuddhi chakra. The spiritual experience created by the element is jnana loka and anandamaya kosha.

VAYU TATTWA – *the element of air.*

Vayu can be translated as air. The element is gray-blue and is symbolized by a hexagon. Vayu stands for kinetic energy in all its forms: electrical, chemical, vital and prana. Its quality is movement and it controls all movement qualities in the body which consist of prana, apana, samana, udana and vyana. Vayu is responsible for our ability to experience physical touch. When we develop the mind for touch, we can experience the feeling of energy in us and around us. Even vayu is physically invisible. The element can be described as "energy in motion". Movement creates change, which means that this element can cause stability and instability both in humans and in the environment. Vayu has its seat between the heart and the eyebrows. Mentally, the element relates to the subconscious mind. Its psychic centers are the Anahata chakra. The spiritual experience of vayu is maha loka and vijnamaya kosha, our intuitive body.

AGNI TATTWA – *the element of fire.*

Agni or fire is known as tejas which means "to sharpen". The element is primarily energy and is experienced as light. With the help of light, we can see the shape. The sense organ that agni relates to is the eye and it gives us the ability to see. Form or matter is the core of the emergence of our ego. The ego identifies with form, which leads to attachment to things. Agni tattwa is thus not only the first manifestation of the form but also the stage when ahamkara begins to grow. The element wears the color red, which indicates fire and heat. The yantra is a red triangle. Agni is often called the "devouring force" and stands for instability. The power of fire is destructive but can be seen as a catalyst for change, developme-

nt and evolution. In our physical body, tattwa agni regulates our digestive fire, appetite, thirst and sleep. It has its place between the heart and the navel. Its psychic centers are the Manipura chakra. The spiritual experience of the element is swar loka and manomaya kosha, our mental / thought body.

APAS TATTWA – *the element of water.*

Apas can be described as a large amount of intensively active matter that has emerged from agni tattwa. It is matter that is not yet coherent as the molecules and atoms are in great chaos. It is said that the universe takes the form of tattwa apas before it appears. Yantra for the element is a horizontal crescent surroun-ded by water. In our physical body, we can see apas in the form of blood, mucus, bile and lymph fluid as it controls our body fluids. The element affects our thoughts related to ourselves and worldly things. The apas has its seat between the navel and the knees. Mentally, it relates to our subconscious and conscious mind. Its psychic centers are the Swadhisthana chakra. The spiritual experience of tattwa apas is bhuvar loka and pranamaya kosha, our energy body.

PRITHVI TATTWA – *the element of earth.*

The last tattwa is prithvi which is also called bhumi, "to be". In prithvi, the motion of the particles has stopped almost completely. Energy has become matter in solid, liquid or gas form. This element bears the yellow color and the yantra is a yellow square. It has the qualities of firmness, weight and cohesion. In our phy-sical body, we can see this in the form of bones and other organs. Since prithvi has emerged from all the other elements, it has all the qualities in itself, but smell is the dominant quality. The element creates stability physically, mentally and in our environment and stands for the material. It has its physical place between our toes and knees. Mentally, it relates to the conscious and subconscious mind. Its psychic centers are the Mooladhara chakra. The spiritual experience of prithvi tattwa is bhu loka and annamaya kosha, our physical body.

TATTWAS AND KOSHAS

The elements build up layers that in yoga are called koshas. Man is said to be made up of five different layers, all of which vibrate differently and relate to different levels of consciousness. The first and coarsest layer is called annamaya kosha which is our physical body and which is made up of food. Pranamaya kosha is the layer of prana, manomaya kosha is the layer of thoughts, vijnamaya kosha is the layer of intuition and the last layer is the layer of body bliss, anandamaya kosha.

These subtle layers of man can only be affected with the help of yoga,tantra and other spiritual exercises. In tattwa shuddhi, annamaya kosha and pranamaya kosha are affected by controlling respiration and increasing the flow of prana. Manomaya kosha is affected by concentration. Vijnamaya kosha is aroused by concentration on tattwa yantras. There is no direct exercise to influence anandamaya kosha. It is necessary to work with the other four layers of bodies to get an experience of anandamaya kosha.

Experiences of color, light and smell that come up during tattwa shuddhi are experiences of our subtle bodies.

Koshas are also linked to seven planes of consciousness. These are called lokas. Each loka relates to a plane of existence through which consciousness develops. The elements have an influence on each loka and through tattwa shuddhi we also influence these.

TATTWAS AND BREATHING

In our physical body, elements such as chitta Shakti, prana Shakti and atma Shakti are manifested. These act in the body and mind through our energy channels, nadis or breathing (swara). Swara and nadi mean flow. Nadi is the flow of Shakti in our subtle body while swara shastra is the flow of our breathing in nadis. Swara shastra is thus the science behind the flow of breathing and nadis. The three Shakti that flow in our breath are channeled through three main nadis in the body (ida, pingala and sushumna). It is said that we have about seventy-two thousand nadis in the body. Ida, pingala and sushumna are responsible for the psychosomatic and spiritual parts of the body, mind and consciousness.

Chitta Shakti, which is the power of ida nadi, is our vital and mental energy that controls all our functions regarding thoughts, mind and chitta. All mental activity is the result of the flow of ida. This flow is connected to our left nostril and affects the right side of the brain. It is also called chandra swara and relates to the negative aspect of the energy in the body.

Prana Shakti flows through the pingala nadi. It is the vital life energy and relates to the positive aspect of it. All physical activity is controlled by prana Shakti. The flow of pingala nadi is connected to our right nostril and affects the left side of the cerebral hemisphere. It is also called surya swara. Atma Shakti is channeled through sushumna nadi. Pranan's central passage for spiritual consciousness. Sushumna is neutral energy and is active when breathing flows through both nostrils at the same time. This condition affects the activity of the dormant parts of the brain. In our physical body, these three nadis relate to the parasympathetic (ida), sympathetic (pingala) and autonomic (sushumna) nervous systems. In most people, sushumna is closed for most of their lives, which means that they are controlled by ida and pingala. Through yogic and tantric exercises, one can open up sushumna nadi.

These three aspects of energy manifest in our breathing cycles. The flow lasts about an hour in each nostril. When the flow changes, the sushumna is open for a few seconds. In our flow of swara, the elements are included. Each element has a specific pranic frequency and affects various bodily functions. Tattwas cause the swara to flow in different directions and affect ida, pingala and sushumna. Ida and pingala nadi channel shakti to the chakras in the body and affect their vibration. The elements also affect the chakras in the body through breathing. Each chakra is dominated by one element – Mooladhara by the earth element, Swadhisthana by the water element, Manipura by the fire element, Anahata by the air element and Vishuddhi by the air element. Just as breathing affects our mental, physical and spiritual existence, so do the elements through their different character affect our state of mind, body and consciousness.

Through various tantric and yogic techniques, it is possible to practice the feeling for which tattwa is active in the swara for the moment. A tattwa yogi can in this way assess his physical, mental, emotional and spiritual condition. Examples of exercises that practice the ability are trataka on tattwa yantras as well as sensations of the elements (color and shape) during the performance of naumukhi mudra, yoni mudra or shanmukhi mudra. The last-mentioned exercises practice our knowledge and experience of the elements as they work. You close the gates for external perception and at the same time open up to the inner experience of color, sound, smell and form.

MANTRA, YANTRA & MANDALA

The theory and philosophy behind tantra are closely intertwined with mantra, yantra and mandala. Tantra is both a philosophical and practical science where its sublime theories become effective through the use of mantra, yantra and mandala. The unique thing about tantra is that there is always an explanation and practical exercise for each philosophy or theory. Mantra, yantra and mandala are used in all tantric exercises. Also within tattwa shuddhi.

MANDALA

The word mandala means circle, and in Hindu and Buddhist rituals it refers to a figure drawn on the ground or painted on a table and symbolizes the cosmic and celestial regions. Mandala is a kind of meditation figure constructed of circles and shapes. Properly depicted and properly inaugurated, it becomes a concentration of occult energy, which attracts hidden forces and itself emits rays like a talisman. Within the boundaries of the mandala circle, other geometric figures are drawn: smaller squares, triangles and circles that divide it all into sacred zones.

To be able to create a mandala, one must be able to see into oneself. Not by thinking – but by vision, as clearly and distinctly as with open eyes. The clearer the inner vision, the more powerful the mandala that is created. The principle behind a mandala is that it exists in the form of a circle. The circle stands for the basic shape behind everything. Anything can shape a mandala, a tree, a house, a car, an animal, or a human being. Even the body is a mandala. To be able to create a mandala that carries strength and power, one must have the ability to create an exact copy of the inner vision. Mandala is the essence of an object experienced by someone who has refined the inner vision, an inner cosmic image of which everyone can partake. The level of consciousness lays the foundation for what the mandala will look like. All forms of art, sculpture and architecture are from the beginning mandala's given form.

In tantra, mandalas are also depicted in the form of illustrated images of divine forces. A human form of the divine makes it easier for the rough mind of man to understand and experience the power within when the ability to visualize is weak. The symbolism and structure behind the images of deities are intended to awaken the equivalent in the consciousness of the individual. By concentrating on mandalas, deeply rooted samskaras are awakened within.

Perhaps the most talked about mandala created in tantra is maithuna kriya. Maithuna kriya forms a mandala that has corresponding yantras and mantras. The erotic sculptures of the Khajuraho Temple in Orissa are based on the tantric belief that maithuna is an act intended to awaken the divine forces in man. The man represents Shiva, the physical energy, and the woman represents Shakti, the mental energy. Through their exoteric and esoteric union, mandalas are created in the form of a force field or energy circle. Linga and yoni mandala are also symbols of this higher union. Man and woman physically unite with each other to re-experience the unity from which they were created. This union is an inner experience in the same way as the spiritual experience.

YANTRA

A yantra is an abstract mathematical image of an inner vision. Behind each rough shape is a subtle shape, which the yantra represents. Everything in nature can be experienced in its original form (yantra). It carries an inherent energy just like everything else in creation. By visualizing and concentrating on the yantra, one can awaken the corresponding energy in oneself. The yantra is made up of the basic and original shapes: a bindu/dot, a circle, a square and a triangle. Bindu is the point from which everything has been created and to which everything will return; it is the process of creation and dissolution. It also represents the union between Shiva and Shakti. Bindu is also found in our physical body, on the top of the back of the head and is called bindu visarga. During meditation, one uses the outer bindu in the form of a yantra, to experience the contraction of time and space in bindu in the physical body. The triangle stands for the first shape that comes out of creation and is also known as the moola tricona (spelling should be trikona in English). Upside down it stands for Prakriti (creation) and with the tip facing upwards, it stands for Purusha (consciousness). The circle represents the cycle of timelessness where neither the beginning nor the end exists, only eternity. This symbolizes the process of birth, life and death. The square is the base on which the yantra rests and represents the physical, earthly world that must be refined.

Yantras create a path from the outer to our inner. They are of great importance for our continued spiritual evolution: they strengthen our creative and intuitive sides, as well as our spiritual experiences. In tattwa shuddhi, one uses yantra created from the four basic forms.

MANTRA

In the same way that every thought has an equivalent in the form of an image, every image also has an equivalent in the form of sound, nada or vibration. These sounds are called mantras. Mantra means "contemplating what leads to liberation". Nada is one of the first manifestations of creation, the form. In Indian philosophy it is believed that the first sound of creation was the sound of "Om" which is the cosmic mantra. Mandukyo Upanishad describes how the mantra affects and expands different levels of consciousness. "Om" is made up of three syllables "A", "U" and "M" which all vibrate at different frequencies which affect the consciousness in different ways. When you repeat "Om", you raise awareness to the same frequency as the mantra. This applies to all mantras.

Nada consists of four frequencies: para (cosmic), pashyanti (temporary), madhyama (subtle) and vaikhari (rough) and correspond to the four frequency levels that "Om" carries: consciously, unconsciously, subconsciously and turya. The entire Sanskrit alphabet consists of mantras. In Sanskrit, the letters are not called letters but akshara, which means imperishable. Each akshara can be used as a mantra. Therefore, it is said that only by reading Vedas can one achieve liberation.

The most powerful form of the mantra is the bija mantra. Bija means seed and is the sound from which all other mantras are derived. The Bija mantra is a powerful, concentrated energy attributed to different levels of consciousness. In tattwa shuddhi, bija mantras are used that relate to the five elements. Even in tantra, it is known that each physical body part has a mantra to which it corresponds. These mantras are used in nyasa to transform the physical body into a container for greater powers, which is aroused by tattwa shuddhi and other esoteric techniques.

Breathing has its mantra created by the sound of inhaling (So) and exhaling (Ham) and is known as the ajapa japa mantra. In the Upanishads it is said that this mantra is powerful enough in itself to be able to awaken Kundalini Shakti and expand consciousness. In the introduction to tattwa shuddhi, the mantra So Ham is used to create a sense of belonging to the universal consciousness.

By repeating the mantra you raise the consciousness, and by concentrating on a yantra you focus the consciousness to a point. At a level of consciousness, the inner experience manifests itself in the form of a thought or emotion, at a higher level it becomes an inner vision or mandala. When you go deeper, it turns into a yantra that is later manifested as sound, nada or mantra. When the mind functions under lower and coarser frequencies of energy, it becomes static, sluggish, slow and tamasic. When you make the energy more subtle through mantra, yantra and mandala, the state of mind changes from tamasic to becoming rajasic and finally sattvic.

Mantras, yantras and mandalas used in tattwa shuddhi have nothing to do with religion, occultism or mysticism. They should be regarded as highly charged forces whose intention is to create the same frequency in man that the mantra, yantra or mandala itself carries to raise consciousness.

VISUALIZATION AND FANTASY

To be able to create, one must first and foremost have the ability to visualize and fantasize. Imagination is a mental ability that can be used in all ways. When you create an inner world of visions and symbols, the power of the mind becomes stronger. In tantra, visualization and imagination create a link between the objective and subjective worlds. Tantric visualizations serve as a guide for the practitioner, a medium to concentrate on. In tattwa shuddhi you want to make the practitioner experience their inner self through the creation of colors, sounds and images, and visualization of these in concrete form. The pictures are both grotesque and pleasant. The practitioner has clear guidelines to follow to help him reach deeper. In the beginning, you experience the images in the form of thoughts, which over time develop into clear, inner images.

THE PERFORMANCE OF PAPA PURUSHA

– the sinful man.

The meditation exercises in tattwa shuddhi consist of many unusual fantasies. The most bizarre of these is papa purusha. Papa purusha symbolizes the cause of suffering, conflict, disharmony and imbalance caused by ego, jealousy, pride, etc. During the exercise, you imagine how papa purusha is transformed and takes shape, which means that you transform yourself. Papa purusha's transformation refers to the inner transformation. The transformation and conflict between the negative and positive forces (ida and pingala) constantly strive to unite and transform into the third neutral force. This conflict acts as a catalyst for our evolution and causes us to continue to seek balance in life. In our search for balance, we turn to the spiritual paths, which guide our evolution further and further forward. Without the conflict between the opposites of energies, we would remain complacent and lazy. Tantra emphasizes the importance of experiencing conflict to create harmony.

The performance of papa purusha is covered on the stage during the exercise when you have become the experience. You witness every action and thought. Each reaction is assessed objectively. It is only then, when one can look at oneself objectively, that one can see the sides of one's personality that the ego has previously hidden; ages you would rather not see or know about. Here, too, Tantra emphasizes the importance of daring to see oneself as one is, not as one wants to be. Only then do you have the opportunity to change yourself?

BHASMA

Tattwa shuddhi includes a symbolic act where one lubricates the body with ash (bhasma) to cleanse the body physically as well as subtly. The great yogi Shiva, who is the father of tantra, is often depicted sitting naked and anointed in ashes. Lubricating oneself with bhasma is considered to favor the experience and discovery of one's own Shiva nature.

Bhasma means "dissolution" or "decomposition" and refers to the decomposition of matter using fire or water. The "bhasmatic" form of matter is produced, which is considered to be a purer and finer form than the original and all impurities disappear. All matter must undergo this process to finally be transformed into the fine essential form. This also applies to us humans. To cleanse means the elimination of slag and impurities. The application of bhasma symbolizes the journey that our inner consciousness makes from rough matter to pure consciousness.

Bhasma is also used in Ayurveda as a medical treatment method. Bhasma can be made of gold, silver, copper or other metals. In tattwa shuddhi, cow dung is used. The use of cow dung in India is common as they are considered antibacterial and antiviral as well as generally beneficial to the skin. The reason why you use cow dung in tattwa shuddhi and no other substance is important. By dis-

solving the cow dung with the help of agni (fire) one reduces it to its bhasmatic form which symbolizes the dissolution of our senses which we try to do in tattwa shuddhi. Through pratyahara we loosen up the experience of the objective world, our surroundings. Through dharana we concentrate the experience of what is left to experience and through dhyana we broaden this experience to its original cosmic essence, the Shiva consciousness.

In tattwa shuddhi, bhasma is applied to the forehead at the same time as the mantra is pronounced, towards the end of the exercise. Most people who have done this experience a feeling of having been deeply cleansed. Rishis and yogis have used bhasma throughout the ages and its beneficial effect has led to the technology being used even today.

THE EFFECT OF TATTWA SHUDDHI SADHANA

The effects of tattwa shuddhi are faster and more powerful when compared to other sadhana, as it is a tantric upasana that one dedicates to Shakti, the energy principle behind everything. The effects manifest themselves both materially and as mental forces (siddhis). However, it is important to keep in mind to perform tattwa shuddhi correctly so as not to create imbalances and obstacles that interfere with the continued spiritual development. It is important to learn the technique from a knowledgeable teacher or guru. Regularity is important for the exercise, not how often you practice. In tantra we want to train the mind, intellect and consciousness. We want to be able to control it with our willpower. To teach us that, regular practice is important.

PHYSICALLY

The combination of fasting and tattwa shuddhi contributes to changes throughout our physical body. When we cleanse the elements (tattwas) that our body is built of, our heart, liver, kidneys, pancreas and all other organs are affected. Tissues and cells are renewed and given new energy, which contributes to a healthier body and mind. Bhasma has a cooling effect on the body and nervous system, which can be heated during intense meditation.

MENTALLY

By visualizing and concentrating on tattwa yantras, chant mantras and creating mandalas, we purify samskaras that can be manifested through dreams, visions and thoughts in our conscious mind. Mental visions are a common effect of most yogic exercises, but within tattwa shuddhi these are usually stronger when one has developed a sharp inner consciousness. You can experience these as subtle sounds, smells, a feeling on the skin, or as taste and shape.

SIDDHIS

Yoga shastras clearly describe that siddhis can be achieved by concentrating on tattwas. By awakening tattwas, one develops higher abilities such as clairvoyance, telepathy and intuition. The elements of the earth help to cure diseases and make the body light. Apas tattwa evens out the flow of prana in the body and enables astral travel. Agni tattwa can turn base metals into precious metals. Vayu tattwa provides knowledge about the past, present and future. Akasha tattwa develops mental projection and reveals metaphysical reality. Despite this, siddhis are not what we strive for in tattwa shuddhi but the purpose is higher spiritual experiences that involve the knowledge of the subtle forces that permeate the entire universe. You thus become more receptive to these forces. You naturally become more intuitive and experience bliss on all levels. In tantric texts, one can also read that the knowledge of the elements leads one to freedom from suffering. This is done through the knowledge that all matter is perishable, and that the human body is the result of atoms, molecules and energy particles. You stop attaching to things and matter when you know what they consist of – ie. composite energy.

TATTWA SHUDDHI

PERFORMANCE

Before you start practicing tattwa shuddhi, you and your teacher/guru should take a sankalpa regarding how long and how often you should practice. It is said that a sankalpa should be as short as one day. The person's willpower and men-

tal ability should be taken into account when determining the time period. A sankalpa must always be completed. You can start practicing at any time during the year, but it is said that the period July-August (shravan) or October (ashwin, the month of devi worship) gives the best results.

You should look after your diet during exercise. Heavy food makes the body sluggish and slow and is difficult for the body to digest and can make it harder to be receptive to higher energies. Salt, strong spices and beverages should be avoided as they increase digestion and can cause too much acid to form. Light foods are preferred such as dairy products, fruits and cooked vegetables. If you have decided to do tattwa shuddhi daily, or for some other reason can not keep a light diet, you should adjust the diet to what is best suited. The special requirements regarding fasting and diet do not need to be followed if one does not have a strict sadhana and only practices tattwa shuddhi once a day.

According to tradition, tattwa shuddhi should be practiced three times a day. During Brahma muhurta (before sunrise), in the afternoon and during sandhya (dusk). Before the exercise, wash yourself. You should practice in a quiet, calm place with few impressions and sit facing north or east. Before the exercise, light a candle and read out your sankalpa. During the last day, practice mouna and after the last completed exercise, sit and meditate on the formless reality.

Step 1: Preparation.

Practice trataka or pranayama for ten to fifteen minutes before the exercise to calm the mind and go deeper into yourself (pratyahara).

Sit in a comfortable meditation position, close your eyes and practice kaya sthairyam.

Visualize the form of your guru or spiritual guide and feel reverence for him/her.

Take your attention to the Mooladhara chakra and imagine how the Kundalini Shakti rises upwards with the sushumna nadi to the Sahasrara chakra on top of the head. Meditate on the mantra So Ham, synchronize with breathing: So on inhalation, from Mooladhara to Sahasrara and Ham on exhalation from Sahasrara to Mooladhara. Experience the movement of the mantra and the breathing as if it were the movement of your inner consciousness.

Step 2: The creation of tattwa yantras.

Take consciousness to the area between the toes and knees. Visualize the shape of a yellow square which is the yantra for prithvi tattwa, the earth's element. Experience its golden yellow color and weight. At the same time, repeat the bija mantra Lam.

Move your attention to the area between the knees and the navel. Visualize a horizontal crescent moon with two white lotus flowers at each end. The crescent is surrounded by a circle of water. This is the yantra of the apas tattwa, the element of water. Repeat with the mantra Vam.
Move the attention further to the area between the navel and the heart. Visualize there a red upside-down triangle burning, which is the yantra for agni tattwa, the element of fire. Simultaneously repeat the mantra Ram.

Now shift your attention to the area between the heart and the eyebrow center. Visualize a hexagon blue in color, which is yantra for the vayu tattwa. Repeat with the mantra Yam.

Move your attention to the area between the center of the eyebrow and the top of the head. Imagine a circle, the yantra of akasha tattwa, the element of space/ ether. In the circle, there is shoonya (the emptiness) and it is black or filled with multicolored dots. Repeat the mantra, Ham.

Step 3: Resolution of the elements.

Take consciousness back to prithvi yantra. Experience how its form becomes fluid and turns into apas, apas into agni, agni into vayu and vayu into akasha.

Now imagine how the aksha is transformed into its origin, the ahamkara, the ego.

The ego is then transformed into the mahat tattwa, the great principle. Mahat tattwa dissolves and becomes Prakriti, Prakriti to Purusha (the highest self). Consider yourself the highest principle, pure and complete.

Step 4: Transformation of the lower nature.

Pay attention to the left side of the abdomen/stomach. Visualize there a small man as big as your thumb. He is called papa purusha. His skin is black as soot, he has glowing eyes and a big belly. In one hand he holds an ax and in the other a shield. He is grotesque in form. You will now transform this man with the help of breathing and mantras.

Hold the right nostril with your right thumb and inhale through the left nostril. At the same time, repeat the mantra Yam four times. Visualize how his face and body transform.

Hold both nostrils. Hold your breath and at the same time repeat the mantra Ram four times. See how the little man is burned to ashes.

Exhale the ashes through your right nostril while repeating the mantra Vam four times. See how the ashes are rolled up into a ball that is mixed with the nectar from the moon in the apas yantra.

Now repeat the mantra Lam. Imagine how the ball on the left side of your stomach transforms into a golden egg.

Repeat the mantra Ham and at the same time visualize how the golden egg grows in size and fills your whole body. It feels like you are born again.

Step 5: Re-formation of the elements.

Reshape the elements in reverse order. From the golden egg, you become again the highest principle, Prakriti, mahat tattwa, ahamkara.

From ahamkara you see how akasha yantra is created, from akasha is created vayu, from vayu is created agni, from agni is created apas, from apas is created prithvi.

Locate the area for each tattwa yantra and repeat the mantra for each tattwa as before.

Step 6: Kundalini back to Mooladhara.

When you have recreated all the elements, repeat the mantra So Ham along with the sushumna synchronized with the breathing. Move the attention from Mooladhara to Sahasrara and from Sahasrara to Mooladhara.

Experience how you, with the separation of jivatma (your soul), separate from paramatma (the cosmic soul). Place jivatma at the heart where its location.

Visualize the Kundalini Shakti that you directed to the Sahasrara and experience how it returns down to the Mooladhara through the sushumna while piercing each chakra on the way down.

Step 7: The shape of the shakti.

Bring your attention to chidakasha. See in front of you a large, deep sea with a large red lotus flower on the water. On the lotus flower see the shape of prana Shakti.

Her body is the same color as a sunrise and decorated with ornaments. She has three eyes and six arms. In her first hand, she holds a trident, in the second a bow made of sugar cane, in the third a snare, in the fourth a spur, in the fifth five arrows, and in the sixth a skull with blood dripping from it.

Keep looking at her beautiful shape and say to yourself" May she give us happiness".

Step 8: Application of bhasma.

Become aware of yourself sitting on the floor. Become body conscious. Inhale slowly and deeply. Open your eyes.

Take some bhasma on the middle and ring fingers and slowly pull the fingers on the forehead from left to right while pronouncing the mantra "Om Hraum Namah Shivaya" or "Om Ham Sa" (Sannyasins).

Take bhasma on your thumb, draw a line from right to left above the other two lines and pronounce the same mantra again.

LESSON NO. 6

LONG SHAVASANA – DEAD MAN'S POSTURE/RELAXATION.

SUPTA PAWANMUKTASANA – THE LEG LOCK.

SHAVASANA – DEAD MAN'S POSTURE.

SURYA NAMASKARA – SUN SALUTATION WITHOUT BREATHING.

SHAVASANA – DEAD MAN'S POSTURE.

VAYU NISHKASANA – THE PUMP.

SHAVASANA – DEAD MAN'S POSTURE.

SHAVA UDARAKARSHANASANA – THE UNIVERSAL POSITION.

SHAVASANA – DEAD MAN'S POSTURE.

BHUJANGASANA – THE COBRA.

SHASHANKASANA – THE HARE.

SHAVASANA – DEAD MAN'S POSTURE.

YOGA NIDRA – DEEP RELAXATION.

KAYA STHAIRYAM & AJAPA JAPA – STEP 1 + 2 + 3 – MEDITATION.

END WITH – HARI OM TAT SAT, 3 TIMES.

THEN – OM SRI DURGAYAI NAMAH, 1 TIME.

INSTRUCTIONS FOR ASANAS LESSON NO. 6

LONG SHAVASANA – DEAD MAN'S POSTURE/RELAXATION.

Execution: See module 1.

SUPTA PAWANMUKTASANA – THE LEG LOCK.

Execution: See module no. 1 & 2.

SHAVASANA – DEAD MAN'S POSTURE.

Execution: See module no. 1 & 2.

SURYA NAMASKARA – SUN SALUTATION WITHOUT BREATHING.

Execution: See module 3.

SHAVASANA – DEAD MAN'S POSTURE.

Execution: See module no. 1 & 2.

VAYU NISHKASANA – THE PUMP.

Execution: See module 3.

SHAVASANA – DEAD MAN'S POSTURE.

Execution: See module no. 1 & 2.

SHAVA UDARAKARSHANASANA – THE UNIVERSAL POSITION.

Execution: See module 1 & 2.

SHAVASANA – DEAD MAN'S POSTURE.

Execution: See module no. 1 & 2.

BHUJANGASANA – THE COBRA.

Execution: See module 2.

SHASHANKASANA – THE HARE.

Execution: See module 1 & 2.

SHAVASANA - DEAD MAN'S POSTURE.

Execution: See module no. 1 & 2.

YOGA NIDRA – DEEP RELAXATION.

Execution: See module 3.

KAYA STHAIRYAM & AJAPA JAPA – STEP 1 + 2 + 3 – MEDITATION

Execution: See module 3.

VISHUDDHI CHAKRA (READ ABOUT THE CHAKRANA IN MODULE 4)

To practice regularly for a month.

Chakra and kshetram localization/activation & purification with Ham chanting. Press one finger against the neck and one finger at the corresponding point on the other side of the neck. Inhale and hold your breath as you experience the pulsation from the chakra and visualize the color while saying Ham silently to yourself. You can also visualize the yantra. Exhale and then continue in the same way for 5-10 minutes.

Ajapa japa with ujjayi pranayama and khechari mudra. See module 3.

KNOWLEDGE TEST MODULE 6

ANSWER AS FULLY AS YOU CAN, THEN CHECK IF YOU ANSWERED CORRECTLY. PRACTICE UNTIL YOU KNOW THE ANSWERS BY HEART.

1. WHAT IS TANTRA?

2. DESCRIBE TATTWA SHUDDHI.

3. DESCRIBE PANCHA TATTWA.

4. DESCRIBE ANTAH KARANA.

5. DESCRIBE MANDALA.

6. DESCRIBE YANTRA.

7. DESCRIBE SIDDHIS.

8. DESCRIBE BHASMA.

9. DESCRIBE VISHUDDHI CHAKRA, ITS ELEMENT, YANTRA, CO-LOR, NUMBER OF PETALS AND ATTRIBUTES.

10. DESCRIBE SOME POWERFUL EXERCISES TO ACTIVATE, CLEAN AND BALANCE VISHUDDHI CHAKRA.

MODULE 7

AYURVEDA. WE STUDY VATA, PITTA, KAPHA & YOGA'S EFFECT ON THE THREE DOSHAS AND AYURVEDIC TREATMENTS

We study Ayurveda and our three doshas – vata, pitta, kapha and how they are affected by yoga and diet. We also familiarize ourselves with basic pulse diagnostics. We read about Ayurvedic treatments such as pancha karma and the importance of sesame oil. We study the Bindu visarga and practice exercises to cleanse, balance and activate chakras. We continue to practice in the role of yoga teacher with lesson no. 7 of 8.

Knowledge test: Answer the questions related to module 7. Practice lesson no. 7 with at least 1 participant and humbly accept feedback from them. Ask questions afterward – how was the pace, did you keep to time, did you speak loudly enough, and how well did you understand the exercises?

According to tradition, the knowledge of yoga is passed on from master to student in descending line. This largely oral tradition means that there may be some differences in interpretation.

AYURVEDA

VATA, PITTA & KAPHA

Ayurveda is an Indian health science with roots in the Vedic tradition. Both yoga and Ayurveda originally came into being as Vedic teachings and are believed to be more than five thousand years old.

Ayur means life and Veda means knowledge – the knowledge/science about life. With the help of Ayurveda, we can learn to live in balance with our life force and our entire divine consciousness.

In Ayurveda, the whole person is treated, not just the sick. When you create balance, you simultaneously release the self-healing forces. Ayurveda develops the health potential we have within us and at the same time expands our consciousness.

Ayurveda and yoga originate from the same tradition and have been practiced together for thousands of years. This is often forgotten resulting in yoga and Ayurveda being taught separately. Both classical yoga and Ayurveda take the whole person into account, physically, mentally and spiritually.

You could say that Ayurveda is a tradition of Vedic knowledge that describes how to heal the body and mind while yoga is a tradition of Vedic knowledge that describes the path to self-insight. Achieving self-insight requires that the body and mind are in balance.

UPAVEDAS

Ayurveda is part of the four upavedas that supplement the four Vedas.

Ayurveda is also closely related to the practice of Veda as it treats various mantras and methods to cure diseases.

The four upavedas are:

1. Ayurveda – knowledge of life.

2. Gandharva veda – knowledge of the role of culture, art and music for spiritual development. For example, there is music for various disease conditions.

3. Dhanur veda – knowledge of the importance of behavior for spiritual development.

4. Sthapatya veda – knowledge of the importance of architecture for spiritual development. This veda is also known as vastu and is reminiscent of feng shui. Feng Shui is a philosophy that practices arranging building structures and objects within living spaces to create balance and energy.

THREE DOSHAS

In Ayurveda, there are three doshas or energy principles which control all life processes both internally and externally. Our entire biological existence is based on the interplay between these three energy principles. Doshas are a combination of the five elements: space, air, fire, water and earth.

The doshas also determine what personality type you are. It is usually said that you have one or two doshas that dominate. According to astrology, it is the influence of the celestial bodies (grahas) during conception that determines which dosha becomes the most dominant in each person. There is dosha type one, dosha type two and dosha type three.

In our yoga practice, it is important to understand how the doshas affect us. When we understand the energy principles and how they affect and interact in and around us, we can take full advantage of the fine yogic techniques to create balance and harmony in our physical and subtle bodies. We can adapt our yoga practice to the needs and personality types that we are in to achieve the best possible results.

In Ayurveda, yoga is used as a basis for maintaining a healthy lifestyle but also as a treatment method for diseases. Asanas, pranayamas and meditation are among the best methods to maintain balance in the doshas.

VATA	PITTA	KAPHA
Space/air.	*Fire/water.*	*Water/soil.*
Movement.	*Combustion.*	*Structure.*
Dry.	*A little oily.*	*Fat/oily.*
Light.	*Light.*	*Heavy.*
Cold.	*Warm/hot.*	*Cold.*
Very fast.	*Fast.*	*Slow.*
Hearing/feeling.	*The eyes.*	*Taste/smell.*
The moon.	*The sun.*	*Earth.*

Vata is kinetic energy in all kinds of ways and the force that allows the other two doshas to move. Vata exists as air in our organs, joints and bones. On a deeper level, vata is the life force within us and the power of thought that moves in our minds. Vata controls the central nervous system, the movements of the heart, the intestines, the lungs, the thought processes and the communication between the mind and the body.

Pitta is responsible for the metabolism and conversion process in the body. In addition to digestion, it also melts our impressions of the outside world, emotions and ideas. Pitta provides us with intelligence, courage and vitality. Without pitta, we lose motivation and sight to reach our goals in life. In nature, you can see pitta in photosynthesis, which is nature's combustion.

Kapha is the one who unites. It is the stable structure that is associated with bone structure, mucous membranes and joints in the body and rocks and mountains in nature. Kapha provides us with emotions and feelings that contribute to love, care, devotion and faith which causes us to both maintain harmony within ourselves and to unite with others.

Vata, pitta and kapha are closely linked and always work together. In every single cell in the body, these three interact. For vata to be in balance, pitta and kapha must exist in the right proportion because it has these two elements in them in the form of water and fire. Vata is the easiest to get out of balance, but it is also the easiest to rebalance. Pitta, in turn, needs to be watered with vata's properties of movement and decomposition (start the fire/dampen the fire) and also kapha's building and preserving properties to keep the fire alive. Kapha needs vata to start the movement and pitta for its stimulus and warming properties. Consequently, we see that none of the doshas can exist without the other; they are all equally important.

RAJAS, TAMAS & SATTVA

Prakriti consists of three varying qualities: rajas, tamas and sattva. Rajas is the active, stimulating and positive force that contributes to change. Tamas is the passive and negative force that keeps the old. Sattva is the neutral and balancing force that harmonizes the positive and the negative. All three energies are necessary for everything that happens, even on the spiritual plane.

Sattva is the light, the love and the life. It is the higher spiritual power that makes us develop our consciousness. Rajas is the passion, the twilight and what changes. It is the vital force that lacks stability. It gives rise to emotional fluctuations such as fear and desire, love and hate. Tamas is the dark, the insensitive, and the dead. It is the lower material force that pulls us down to unconscious-

ness, stagnation, listlessness and heaviness. Unmanifested Prakriti keeps these three in balance. Rajas and tamas get sattva together. When Prakriti is manifested, these qualities are distinguished.

Sattva gives rise to the mind, rajas generates the life force and tamas stands for form and substance as the physical body. Yoga and Ayurveda want to develop the sattvic state. In yoga, sattva is the higher quality that makes us develop spiritually. In Ayurveda, sattva is the state of balance in which the healing property is released.

YOGIC AND AYURVEDIC DIET

In Ayurveda, diet plays a very big role and lays the foundation for all other therapeutic approaches and healing processes. Without a proper and balanced diet, other medicines have no major effect. The food is used as medicine. A sattvic diet is advocated because sattva creates balance. A sattvic diet is traditionally based on ahimsa, which is an ethical principle of not causing harm to other living beings. The food should, as far as possible, have been allowed to grow naturally in a harmonious environment as such food carries a lot of prana and pure awareness.

Yogis around the world are usually very aware of what they are eating but a traditional yogic diet and an Ayurvedic one are different. Ayurveda wants to create balance and build good physical health. In yoga, you want to develop and change body awareness. In short: Ayurveda wants to create physical health and yoga helps us to get beyond the limits of the body. Many traditional yogic paths are ascetic where solid, simple raw foods with detoxifying effects are common. However, these have a water-raising effect. Traditional Ayurvedic diet is instead based on well-cooked and nutritious food to strengthen us physically and prevent any of the doshas from becoming unbalanced and or unnecessarily wet.

A traditional yogic diet increases the elements of space/ether and air(vata) to detoxify and open up the mind. Therefore, raw food and fasting are recommended. By reducing the body, you expand the mind. Another significant factor in the yogic diet is prana. A raw diet is rich in prana. By following a raw diet, you increase the flow of prana in the body and thus purify nadis. Breathing exercises are used to increase the digestive fire in the body, which allows the food to be digested even though it's not cooked.

However, few of us can digest this type of food satisfactorily. This is especially true for vata people who have varying digestive fire, but even kapha and pitta can have difficulty with this. Therefore, most non-ascetics feel better from a well-cooked, warm diet that is easy to digest.

An Ayurvedic diet is not necessarily sattvic but is more focused on creating physical health. A Yogic diet, on the other hand, places the greatest emphasis on the food's satiety, which can increase a dosha. For an optimal diet, you can choose sattvic food that is adapted to your dominant dosha type. Sattvic food includes dairy products, natural oils, herbal teas, sweet spices, fruits, fresh juices, vegetables, cereals, legumes, nuts, seeds and honey. For a sattvic diet, it is important to eat the right type of food at the right time during the day because the day is also divided into vata, pitta and kapha time. In Ayurveda, it is recommended to eat light food for breakfast because Kapha time prevails and heavy food weighs down the mind and body as well. The biggest goal should be to eat in the middle of the day during pitta time when digestion is at its strongest. In the evening, you should not eat heavy foods or too close to bedtime as it disturbs both sleep and the natural cleansing of waste materials.

THE SIX TASTES

Six different flavors affect each dosha in different ways. Each flavor consists of a combination of two elements.

Sweet – water and soil.
Balances vata and pitta. Increases kapha. For example, vegetables, oils, milk and rice.

Sour – fire and soil.

Balances vata. Increases pitta and kapha. For example, citrus, yogurt, cheese and vinegar.

Salt – fire and water.

Balances vata. Increases pitta and kapha. For example, seaweed, tamari, table salt.

Pungent – fire and air.

Decreases kapha. Increases pitta and vata. For example, strong spices such as pepper, onion and ginger.

Bitter – space and air.

Balances pitta and kapha. Increases vata. For example, green leafy vegetables and turmeric.

Astringent – air and soil.

Balances pitta and kapha. Increases vata. For example, beans, lentils and unripe bananas.

TIP

Try to eat in silence and a relaxed manner. Focus on the meal and not on anything else at the same time. Eat foods you like and avoid cold foods. Avoid eating when you feel anxious, angry or sad. Drink boiled water with food, not milk. Eat freshly prepared food as much as possible and avoid leftovers, as the nutrients have already been lost. The food must be prepared with love and awareness.

AGNI

In Ayurveda, the body's digestive fire – called agni, is of great importance. If the fire is too weak, the food cannot be digested satisfactorily and nutrients are lost. The food we eat then instead turns into ama (slag products) which strains our bodies. In Ayurveda, a weak digestive fire is seen as the root cause of most dis-

eases. Our modern life and the stress we live with are major contributing factors to poor digestion. We tend to gulp down food instead of enjoying it.

When we have a balance between the doshas, the agni will also be in balance. A sign of this is when we feel a healthy appetite at regular times.

The agni is weakened when we overeat, snack or eat even though we are not hungry. Refrigerated food, long fasting and poorly chewed food are also contributing factors.

When vata is increased, digestion becomes irregular. It can change from fast to slow and sometimes you can feel a strong hunger and sometimes nothing at all. Stomach problems are also part of the picture.

When pitta gets out of balance, the agni becomes too strong. You may experience a very strong hunger, often shortly after eating. This contributes to nutrients not being absorbed by the body and in the long run you can suffer from stomach ulcers.

When kapha is elevated, digestion becomes very slow instead. You experience a heavy feeling after eating and feelings of hunger are weak.

AGNI YOGA

Both yoga and Ayurveda carry the knowledge of the divine fire, the agni. We learn to control the fire to create balance and to develop. The cosmic fire exists everywhere; in ourselves and around us. In the body, we see the agni in the form of our digestive fire, and on a finer level, the agni corresponds to our eternal consciousness. Without fire, our development and evolution will stop.

In Ayurveda, we learn to balance the function of the agni physically by taking care of our digestive fire, which then lays the foundation for good health. In yoga the focus is on the pranic agni and the fire of meditation, both of which are important for our path to enlightenment. Various fire rituals are common in yoga traditions, but we may be most familiar with the Breath of Fire exercise, which cleanses the body's energy channels and increases the flow of prana in the body.

YOGAS IMPACT ON OUR THREE DOSHAS:

ASANAS AND AYURVEDA

Asanas release tension and energy blockages that may have occurred, thereby keeping the body's tissues, joints and organs in the best possible shape. The positions stretch and strengthen the muscles, and the spine is kept flexible, making it possible for the energy to flow freely through nerves that belong to our organs and glands. Our tissues are therefore cleansed in a systematic way, which prepares the body for more advanced yogic exercises.

Asanas prepare you for breathing exercises and meditation. They not only have a physical purpose but they also affect us on a practical, mental and spiritual level. Asanas have from the beginning aimed to counter rajas, the turbulent energy within us that distracts the mind.

Asanas help to balance and release the prana in the body, which prepares us for breathing exercises. Our senses are turned inward which facilitates mind control (pratyahara). When our thoughts are still, the mind is calmed so that we can concentrate (dharana) and meditate (dhyana).

Diet and asanas are the two most important factors in creating good health and, in the long run, counteracting imbalances and diseases.

To balance the prana in the body, spices, herbs and various breathing exercises are used. To enable this, a proper posture and diet are required as a basis. Our posture is of great importance for our health and consciousness. The body and the mind influence each other through subtle channels in the body through which foods and our thoughts flow. The channels are held together by the musculoskeletal system, the shape of which is determined by our posture. Improper posture causes stress in the body and blocks these channels. The energy cannot flow optimally and residual products and toxins get a chance to accumulate. This eventually leads to discomfort in the body, pain and illness.

It is easy for asanas to become the mainstay of yoga practice. If you want to take part in yoga on a deeper level, you should give equal time to asanas, pranayamas and meditation. An exaggerated and unconscious execution of asanas leads to a fixation on the body and boosts our physical ego: this leads to a rigid and undeveloped mind and emotions. Never exaggerate the exercises or force the body into a position, which will only cause more tension and injury.

ASANAS AND OUR AGE

Infants and children are by nature soft and flexible in the body. Starting to practice asanas at an early age means that you maintain the softness and correct posture for life.

At the age of sixty–five–which is the vata age, the body fluids slowly begin to decrease and dry out. The body becomes stiffer and joint diseases are common. With the help of asanas, you can keep your body in shape and balance excess vata.

Vinyasas are suitable for younger people because a lot of rajas prevail in body and mind and they need vinyasas to mature. After the age of twenty-four, one should move on to inner yoga and develop the mind by studying yogic texts. After the age of forty-eight, the mind develops at the same speed as the physical energies are withdrawn. You should spend more time meditating but asanas are still important for keeping the body supple and healthy.

At the age of seventy-two, the mind develops even more. This is the time for deep meditation. Asanas continue to be important to slow down aging.

ASANAS FOR VATA

Vata people often have a slim and thin physique. They are very flexible and mobile when young but easily develop stiffness as they age. Vatas often suffer from joint problems in middle age. They are often cold, have dry skin, cracked joints, and poor blood circulation. Vata people are naturally nervous and scared, which makes them tense in their shoulders and back. Asanas are very important for vata people, for both their health and their ability to meditate. Vatas must exercise caution when practicing asanas as they are prone to injury. Soft, flowing exercises at a reasonable speed are preferred.

Mental preparation is important for vatas: a moment of rest and deep breathing before asanas is a must. During the actual practice, vatas should start slowly so the circulation awakens and the joints have a chance to warm up. Vatas should not be too sweaty as they dry out easily. Intake of fluid is important. Asanas should mainly affect the area around the hips and intestines which is the main seat of vata. Releasing tension from the hips and lumbar spine is important. Too much stretching and movement can cause over-stretching and weakness.

Sitting positions are good for vata such as padmasana and vajrasana. These have a calming, grounding effect and control apana vayu.

Keeping the spine flexible is important for vatas who often accumulate tension here. Exercises that rotate the spine in each direction are good. Matsyendrasana is an example of a pose that releases vata from the nervous system. It is important to have proper breathing when performing spinal rotation, otherwise, the pose will have the opposite effect and increase vata.

Forward bending positions have a calming effect and release vata from the back. Combining forward bending positions with backward bending positions is important to maximize the benefits. However, this should be done slowly and carefully. Doing backward bending positions too quickly can stimulate the sympathetic nervous system and our "fight or flight" mechanism. With caution, asanas such as the cobra and the grasshopper have a grounding and strengthening effect on vatas.

Standing poses are very good for vata. They build strength, give peace and increase stability.

Vatas should avoid becoming too exhausted. Dynamic asanas should be accompanied by sitting positions in combination with pranayamas and meditation.

After asanas, vatas should lie and rest in shavasana. It is an optimal time to meditate, with the mind calm and the emotions stable.

Seated poses:
Siddhasana/siddha yoni asana (perfect pose), vajrasana (diamond pose) and simhasana (lion pose).

The sun salutation:
Slowly and consciously.

Standing poses:
Vrksasana (tree pose), trikonasana (triangle pose), virabhadrasana (warrior pose), parighasana (gate pose) and all standing forward bending positions.

Inverted poses:
Shirshasana (headstand), vipareeta karani asana (half shoulder stand).

Backbends:
Bhujangasana (cobra) and shalabhasana (grasshopper).

Forward bends:
All. Especially janu sirsasana (half-butterfly) and pachimottasana (pliers).

Spinal twists:
*Lying positions, bharadvajasana (half turn) and shava udarakarshanasana
(universal position).*

Other:
*Shashankasana (hare), parivrtta janu sirsasana (one-legged forward bend in a
seated position), navasana (boat), yoga mudra.*

Shavasana:
At least twenty minutes.

ASANAS FOR PITTA

*Pittas have a medium-sized physique. They often have good muscles and flexibil-
ity. Circulation and joint mobility are usually good due to the slightly oily nature
of pittas. Pittas usually handle asanas very well, but if overdone, it may lead to
hypermobility and stiffness in joints.*

*Mentally, pitta people are aggressive and like to shine in everything they do.
Pittas must be careful about "performing" when it comes to asanas. They can
often become very good at the technical part but forget about the spiritual part.
Pittas are often overambitious, annoyed and very driven. Asanas should be used
to cool pittas down both physically and mentally, thereby helping them turn their
intelligence inward to better understand themselves.*

*Calm breathing and sitting still after powerful asanas are important to counter-
act any stress. Pittas should avoid overly strenuous exercise and not get too hot.
Powerful asanas are ok as long as pittas compensate by using cooling asanas and
pranayamas to cool the mind and body towards the end.*

Around the navel, heat is created and distributed throughout the body. In the palate where saliva is secreted, we have a cooling function in the body. The heat from the umbilical region moves upwards to reduce the cold produced in the soft palate. By standing in a shoulder position or entering the plow position, the cooling property is protected from heat. These positions reverse the positions of the sun and the moon in the body, which creates balance, especially in pitta people. Spinal twists such as matsyendrasana are also good for protecting the cooling property without lowering the fire in the body. Positions that release tension and affect the abdominal tract, small intestine and liver are also beneficial for pittas because pitta accumulates in these areas. The bow, cobra, boat and fish poses are good. Headstand increases pitta and should be avoided if you do not know how to balance the heat afterward.

Forward bending positions are generally good for pittas because they increase the energy around the abdomen, and have a cooling effect and also a grounding effect. Back-bending positions create more heat and should therefore be practiced in moderation and followed by cooling asanas. Seated spinal twists help cleanse the liver and detoxify the pitta.

After asanas, pitta should feel calm, cool and relaxed in the stomach. The mind should be in a meditative state and not too sharp.

Seated poses:
Most are beneficial except simhasana(the lion) which should be avoided.

The moon greeting:
Cooling for pitta.

Standing poses:
Vrksasana (tree pose), trikonasana (triangle pose), ardha chandrasana (crescent pose).

Standing poses(legs wide apart):
Moordhasana(head on the floor from standing with legs apart), padottana-
sana(leg lift).

Forward bends:
All seated forward bends are good, especially pada prasar paschimottanasana
(forward bend with legs split), kurmasana (turtle) and paschimottanasana
(pliers).

Twists:
Ardha matsyendrasana (half spinal rotation).

Other:
Sarvangasana (shoulder stand), vipareeta karani (half shoulder stand), navasa-
na (boat), ardha matsyendrasana (seated spine twisting), bhujangasana (cobra),
yoga mudra.

Shavasana:
Medium, long.

ASANAS FOR KAPHA

Kapha types are heavily built and gain weight easily. They are often inflexible
and should not try to push the body into a position like a lotus position, which
carries a risk of injury. Kapha's body and joints often do not support these po-
sitions. Kaphas must accept how they are built and not try to become thin slim
yogis because their body is not built that way.

Kapha women can be thin when they are young but gain weight over the years,
especially after giving birth. This can weigh down kaphas as they may have a
hard time accepting this. It is then common in this case for them to use different
ways to try to lose weight such as yoga although it rarely gives results. Kaphas
must instead work on their attitude toward their body and accept what is

natural for them. It is important for kaphas to still try to maintain normal body weight without starving themselves.

Obesity in kapha is mainly seen on the abdomen and thighs causing various problems with posture. Increased kapha also causes mucus formation around the breasts and lungs, which then spreads to different parts of the body and causes blockages in the ducts. These blockages contribute to increased fat accumulation around joints and tissues.

Kapha people are rarely physically active, although needing it to stimulate their metabolism and increase circulation. As kaphas are easily affected by high cholesterol and heart disease, they should exercise with caution and be mindful not to overwork while still challenging themselves.

As heat triggers the flow in kaphas, exercises that increase heat and make the body sweat are good. Kaphas need to be pushed to do exercises that are difficult and that they do not think they can do.

Sitting asanas increase kapha. Pranayamas that increase heat are beneficial before meditation.

Vinyasas such as the sun salutation are good to start the flow. Backward bending positions are also good as they open up the chest, which is the area for kapha. Backbends also increase circulation in the head, which counteracts inertia. Forward bending positions should generally be avoided by kaphas unless they need to calm the nervous system.

Kaphas often suffer from slow digestion. Exercises, like the arch, that initiate the flow at the navel region are therefore particularly good. The plow is one of the best positions to open up the lungs. Pranayamas initiate the flow in both body and mind.

After asanas, kaphas should feel light and warm and have increased circulation in the body. Chest and lungs should be open and the mind should feel clear and alert.

Seated poses:
Simhasana (the lion) and in combination with pranayamas.

The sun salutation:
At a fast pace.

Standing poses:
Virabhadrasana (warrior), Utthita hasta padangusthasana (hand-to-toe stand), bakasana (crow), ardha chandrasana (crescent position).

Inverted poses:
Adho mukha vrksasana (downward facing dog) sirsasana (head stand), sarvangasana (shoulder stand).

Backbends:
Ustrasana (camel pose), shalabasana (grasshopper pose).

Other:
Shava udarakarshanasana (spinal rotation), ardha matsyendrasana (half spinal rotation), parvatasana (mountain pose), halasana (plow pose).

Shavasana:
Short.

PRANAYAMAS
Yoga teaches us how to master prana and thus gain access to its deeper powers. When we learn that, we are no longer in need of external pleasure. In this way, we take control of our mind and can heal it and our body. A knowledgeable

Ayurveda doctor knows how to redirect the prana in the body to heal the patient. In the same way that food, herbs and other healing ways are used to influence the prana.

Pranayama is one of the most central exercises in yoga and is the fourth step in classical yoga. The prana cleanses and revitalizes the body before meditation.

With breathing exercises, you slow down and prolong your breath. This causes the life energy – the prana, to manifest itself.

Breathing exercises have a good effect on diseases that affect the respiratory organs, circulation and nervous system as well as fatigue and a weak immune system. The whole body is affected by the exercises by massaging the internal organs. The circulation increases in the internal organs and is detoxified. Pranayamas also have a good effect on depression, stress and tension.

PRANA AND APANA

The apana associated with gravity moves downwards and results in disease, aging, death and unconsciousness. Prana associated with the elements of air and space moves upwards through our senses. By bringing these two energies together, we can strengthen our energy and awaken our higher abilities. Yogic exercises involve redirecting the apana upwards so that it meets the prana and pulling the prana down so that it meets the apana. This takes place at the solar plexus which is the seat of the prana.

Prana – inhalation.
Samana – hold your breath/contract.
Vyana – hold your breath/expand.
Udana – exhale/squeeze out.
Apana – exhale/elimination.

PRANAYAMA AND PRANA AGNI

Pranayamas develop the fire of prana which is responsible for the body's combustion. This is done by holding your breath. Oxygen acts as food for pranaagni. The carbon dioxide that accompanies the exhalation is its residual product. Holding our breath cleanses our subtle body in the same way that fasting cleanses our physical. Prana agni gives power to Kundalini so it can continue its journey upwards and take with it prana and apana.

PRANAYAMAS AND DOSHAS

Pranayamas affect all doshas. Done correctly, they help balance vata, reduce kapha and counter pitta. Inhalation relates to kapha and has a constructive effect. Holding the breath in relates to the pitta and has a transforming effect. Exhalation relates to vata and has a reducing effect.

Breathing through the right nostril gives power to the pingala nadi and increases pitta. Breathing through the left nostril gives power to ida nadi and increases kapha. Balanced breathing through both nostrils balances vata.

Kapha increases when you breathe through your mouth, which is generally advised against. However, there are some specific breathing exercises where you apply breathing through the mouth which can help the prana to be retained in the sushumna nadi.

VATA

Breathing through the right nostril is revitalizing for vata. Practice with intent in the morning for about ten to fifteen minutes. Breathing through the left nostril has a calming effect and calms the mind. Practice with intent in the evening to improve night sleep. Bhastrika can help with energizing and clarifying the mind but should be done carefully. End the exercise if dizziness occurs.

PITTA

Cooling pranayamas are best suited for pittas. Breathing through the left nostril is beneficial in the evening and in cases of feeling overheated or irritated. Shitali and sitkari pranayamas have a good effect on strong overheating, irritation and emotions.

KAPHA

Breathing through the right nostril is well suited for the morning as it reduces kapha. Bhastrika and kapalbhati are excellent for kaphas, especially for countering the effects of colds (not fever), listlessness and depression.

MEDITATION

Meditation consists mostly of dharana (concentration), dhyana (meditation) and samadhi (ecstasy). These three steps belong to the inner aspect of the eight steps of yoga. In Ayurveda, meditation is used for therapeutic purposes, mainly to heal the mind and psychological diseases but its effect also affects our physical body as our physical body is also affected by our mental state. To be able to meditate, the body, the prana and the senses must be in balance.

Both the body and the mind are made up of the five elements. The body is composed of elements heavy in character such as earth and water (kapha), which shapes our body. The body's functions consist of slightly lighter elements and doshas. Pitta (fire) is responsible for transformations within the body, while vata (air) is responsible for the impulses between our brain and nerve impulses. The mind is made up of the lighter form of vata (air and ether), which makes it volatile. The mind's functions consist of the heavier elements: fire, water and earth (pitta and kapha). Fire provides the mind with perceptions, the water adds emotions and the earth connects the mind with the body. The mind is fast and in perpetual change.

Vatas are more quick-witted than other dosha types. It is easier for them to make new acquaintances (air) and be open to new experiences (ether). Vatas have very active senses and are always on the move somewhere. They are more often affected by mental and psychological imbalances.

Pitta is seen as the insightful part of the mind with the third eye of the mind relating to the element of fire. The fire of the mind is what is called buddhi (intellect and insight). Pitta types are often very intelligent with a good ability to focus and have sharp and clear thinking.

Kaphas feel emotions, love and devotion which are linked to our senses and the external character of the mind (manas). Bliss as the core of the mind is the highest form of kapha.

Meditation allows us to come in contact with our higher self and consciousness (atman and purusha). With the help of meditation, we can cleanse our subconscious from things that cause us suffering. Regardless of the meditation technique used, the purpose is to create the original stillness of our consciousness which is our true nature.

Meditation can help with:
– Psychological diseases.
– Difficulty falling asleep.
– Emotional disorders.
– Chronic diseases such as allergies and asthma that are affected by stress and hypersensitivity in the nervous system.
– Heart disease. According to ancient Vedic texts, our consciousness belongs to the heart. Calming the mind and strengthening the heart, therefore, go hand in hand.
– Pain relief by e.g. focusing on a mantra.
– Preparing for death and leaving the body.

MEDITATION FOR VATA

Meditation can help vatas with their hypersensitive and active mind to: provide better sleep, improve metabolism and strengthen the immune system. Caution must be exercised as meditation performed incorrectly can have the opposite effect on vatas and cause feelings of volatility. Vatas should first and foremost exercise their ability to concentrate. Techniques that include mantras and visualization are good because they saturate the mind instead of "emptying" it. Vatas should not try to calm the natural flow of thoughts but instead observe it and let it flow.

Preparation:
- Relaxing asanas help vata types sit for longer periods.
- Deep breathing exercises increase concentration by providing the body with prana.

Visualizations:
- Earth, fire and water.
- Mountains, lakes, flowers, fire and sunset.

Balancing colors:
- Gold and saffron help vata types achieve mental clarity.

Mantras:
- Ram, Shrim and Hrim.
During meditation or when vata seems to be out of balance.

Deities to meditate on:
- Durga and Tara give a feeling of security.
- Shiva and Vishnu give a feeling of security.
- Ganesha creates a sense of grounding.

Considering vata's anxious and fearful nature, devotion to a god or devotion to any teacher or guru is suitable. In this way, vatas can leave their worries and problems to someone else and get help and experience security at the same time.

Vatas need to learn to experience contact with the eternal within itself, create stability and not worry about the changing world. Vatas need space, peace and *quiet to get away from the pace of their surroundings. Meditation on the true eternal helps to slow down one's thoughts.*

MEDITATION FOR PITTA

Pitta people need meditation to release emotions such as aggression and anger. They often have a good ability to concentrate and it is easy for them to meditate. Mantra meditation is a great way for pittas to take advantage of their strong mental energy by focusing it on a goal. Pitta types must work to expand their mind and heart with the help of the inner light and thus gain insight into the truth. The meditation should provide stillness in the mind and heart of the pitta.

Preparation:
– Soothing asanas that do not create too much heat in the body.
– Shitali pranayama or breathing through the left nostril to cool the system.

Visualizations:
– Mountains, forests, lakes and seas.
– Rain clouds, flowers in cold colors, the moon and the stars.

Balancing colors:
– White, dark blue and green.

Affirmations:
– Devotion, love and forgiveness to balance the fire.
– Prayers for peace and love for other people.
Mantras:
– Shrim, Sham and Om. Recited silently.

Deities to meditate on:
– Lakshmi, Uma parvati, Shiva and Vishnu.

Pittas can be very critical and judgmental. They can use and transform this power by redirecting it to explore their inner self and expand their consciousness. Meditating on infinite space beyond all limitations is beneficial to their critical minds.

MEDITATION FOR KAPHA

Kaphas need meditation to free themselves from old emotional and mental patterns, and to counteract inertia. Kaphas need a lot of encouragement and motivation to meditate so group meditation is usually best suited for them.

It is easy for kaphas to fall asleep and daydream so choosing an active form of meditation can help prevent this from happening. A combined form of meditation and activity with mantras or pranayamas is good.

Preparation:
– Powerful asanas that start the circulation in the body.
– Bhastrika pranayama or breathing through the right nostril.

Visualization:
– Fire, air and ether.
– Sun, wind, sky.

Balancing colors:
– Gold, blue and orange.

Affirmations:
– Which strengthens the connection to the higher self.
For example. "In my true self, I am independent and free, in nature and space."

Mantras:
– Om, Hum and Aim.
Cleansing and stimulating, to be recited out loud.

Deities to meditate on:

– Shiva and Kali. Divinities of an angry nature release emotions and reduce the ego.

Meditating on emptiness and the inner light creates more space and fire in the mind, which is beneficial for kaphas.

PULSE DIAGNOSTICS

In Ayurveda, various techniques are used to establish a diagnosis of one's health. These include analysis of heart rate, urine, feces, eyes, tongue, speech, skin, shape, and most importantly, pulse. Taking one's pulse as a diagnostic tool has been used in Ayurveda since time immemorial. A well-experienced Ayurvedic physicist can use the pulse to assess prakruti (one's general constitution), vikruti (current imbalances in the doshas), subtle imbalances and other diseases.

You can read the pulse in different places in the body – e.g. in the armpit, ankle and wrist, of which the latter is the most common. This is done by placing the index finger, middle finger and ring finger on the upper side of the wrist (towards the thumb). The three fingers represent the three different doshas vata, pitta and kapha. The index finger represents the vata dosha, the middle finger the pitta dosha, and the ring finger the kapha dosha. Each dosha has a characteristic pulse: from where the pulse starts, where on the finger it beats the strongest, from which direction it beats, and what quality the pulse has. Rishis use animal movement patterns to describe heart rate levels:

The vata pulse's movement pattern can be compared to how a cobra moves. It is fast, weak, cold, thin and disappears with pressure and is best felt under the index finger.

The pitta pulse's movement pattern can be compared to a frog. It is prominent, strong, warm, and powerful, lifts the palpating finger and is best felt under the middle finger.

The kapha pulse's movement can be likened to a swimming swan. It is deep, slow, wide, wavy, dense, cold or hot, regular, and can be best felt under the ring finger.

THE SEVEN LEVELS OF THE PULSE

In Ayurveda, the pulse is divided into seven different levels, each of which tells us how we feel mentally, physically and spiritually. You can read the different levels by placing three palpating fingers on the wrist and changing the pressure. The pulses provide the practitioner with vikruti (imbalances) that are present in our doshas at the moment. Manas vikruti (manas: mind).

Subdoshas.
Each dosha(vata, pitta and kapha) has five subdoshas. Each sub dosha represents a particular aspect of our physiology. In each sub dosha, one of the five elements is prominent.

Vata subdoshas: prana, udana, samana, vyana and apana.

Pitta subdoshas: pachaka, ranjaka, alochaka, sadhaka and bharajaka.

Kapha subdoshas: kledaka, avalambaka, bodhaka, tarpaka and shleshaka.

Prana, tejas and ojas. Prana is the essence of vata, tejas is the essence of pitta and ojas is the essence of kapha. Ojas are created during nutrition and are the main essence of all tissues. Tejas can be compared to hormones and amino acids. Prana, which is the vital life energy, is responsible for the cooperation between cells.

Dhatus represents our biological tissues such as plasma, blood tissues, muscle tissues, adipose tissues, bones, nerve tissues, and male and female reproductive tissues.

Prakruti represents our basic psychosomatic and biological constitution. Manas

Prakruti (manas: sun). If a person says that they are, for example, a pitta person, they are not talking about any imbalance but about their basic constitution.

CHINESE MEDICINE

Pulse diagnostics is also an important part of Chinese medicine. However, Ayurvedic pulse diagnostics and Chinese differ somewhat. In Chinese technology, one can read forty-seven different aspects of the pulse, compared with the seven levels present in Ayurveda.

AYURVEDIC TREATMENTS

In Ayurvedic treatment, there are eight main disciplines, so-called ashtangas:

Internal medicine (kaya-chikitsa).
Pediatrics (kaumarabhrityam).
Surgery (shalya-chikitsa).
Eyes (shalakya-tantra).
The science of demonic obsession (bhuta-vidya). Has been called psychiatry.
Toxicology (agada-tantram).
Disease prevention, immunity enhancement and rejuvenation (rasayana).
Aphrodisiacs and improving the health of the offspring (vajikaranam).

AYURVEDIC MASSAGE

Ayurvedic massage is used to treat a variety of diseases and for preventive purposes.

There are at least forty different types of Ayurvedic massage which, along with a variety of other diagnostic tools, are used by Ayurvedic doctors to treat diseases and ill health.

Ayurvedic massage relieves pain, relaxes stiff muscles, reduces swelling caused by joint inflammation, improves blood circulation, increases stress resistance, provides better sleep, increases athletic performance and provides emotional benefits. With Ayurvedic massage, deeply rooted toxins are released in joints and tissues and then eliminated through natural processes.

ABHYANGA – AYURVEDIC OIL MASSAGE

Abhyanga (oil massage) is a common Ayurvedic massage. Abhyanga is a therapeutic massage of about forty-five minutes and is used to treat a large number of diseases. Abhyanga is often given by two therapists working on either side of the client, who is lying on a wooden bed. Particular attention is paid to the feet because there are marma points (nerve nodes) on the soles of the feet that are closely related to certain internal organs. The sole of the right foot is massaged with clockwise movement and the left foot is counterclockwise.

During treatment, the client rests in seven standard positions. Abhyanga begins with the client sitting in an upright position, after which she lies flat on her back, turns to the right side, lies on her back again, turns to the left side, lies on her back again and finally returns to a sitting position. Abhyanga is an essential part of pancha karma therapy.

SHIRO ABHYANGA – AYURVEDIC HEAD MASSAGE

Shiro abhyanga is a head massage with roots in Ayurveda. The purpose of Shiro abhyanga is not only to ward off stress but also to stimulate the body to heal itself. Various oils are usually included as a natural part of the treatment, to soothe the soul and care for the skin and hair. Shiro abhyanga is a head massage which, in addition to Ayurvedic contexts, is common in hair salons in India.

NASYAM – AYURVEDIC NASAL TREATMENT

Nasyam is an Ayurvedic treatment in which medicinal oils are administered through the nose to clear the throat, nose and head of harmful substances. This treatment is used to treat migraines, headaches, mental disorders, prematurely graying hair and speech difficulties. Nasyam is also said to strengthen the mind and intellect and is included in pancha karma treatment.

PANCHA KARMA

Perhaps the most famous form of Ayurvedic treatment is pancha karma. Pancha karma, or literally "five actions" in Sanskrit, is a cleansing treatment to increase the metabolic process with an appropriate diet, natural herbs and minerals. Pancha karma is used both for deep-rooted chronic diseases and for seasonal imbalances of the three elemental energies (doshas) pitta, vata and kapha. The purpose of the treatment is to make the body healthy by eliminating bodily waste products and achieving a balance between the doshas.

Pancha karma – five actions in three steps.

The five measures consist of nasyan (nasal treatment), vamana (vomiting), virechana (detoxing), nirooha vasti (enemas with herbal decoctions), and sneha vasti (enemas with herbal oils). After these treatments, hopefully the body has been cleansed of accumulated toxins.

Panchakarma is always performed in three stages: purva karma (pre-treatment), pradhana karma (primary treatment) and paschat karma (post-treatment). The patient who chooses any of the five treatments above must always undergo all three stages for the treatment to have the intended effect.

Step 1. Pre-treatment (purva karma).
Snehana (oil therapy) is an important preparatory treatment. Snehana is said to loosen toxins that are stuck in different places in the body and are often given with adapted herbal mixtures to treat an individual disease, but can also be given in a pure form without additives. Snehana is given early in the morning for a maximum of seven days and is said to help the transfer of toxins to the gastrointestinal tract so that they can be easily removed afterward. If snehana is not given before pancha karma, the intended effect on the treatment will not be obtained.

Oil massage (abhyanga) is another important treatment in pancha karma.

Svedana is a therapy that induces sweating and is administered to the whole body or parts of the body depending on the disease. Steam with added medicinal herbs is usually used, but can also be achieved by having the patient sit under the sun, while thirsty, hungry, and having their body covered with thick sheets; or by staying in a closed dark room. Svedana is said to dilate ducts in the body and thus helps move toxins to the gastrointestinal tract.

Step 2. Primary treatment (pradhana karma).
The toxins and slag products that reach the gastrointestinal tract are believed to be eliminated during the primary treatment.

One of the five primary treatments, vamana karma, is used for kapha diseases such as bronchitis, colds, coughs, asthma, sinusitis, and excess mucus. One to three days before vamana karma, one is treated with oil both internally and ex

ternally. Externally through abhyanga (Ayurvedic massage) and internally with ghee (shredded butter) in the diet.

Step 3. Post-treatment (paschat karma).
The finishing treatment consists of adapted diets, appropriate physical effort and intake of herbs to promote long-term health.

AYURVEDA AND SESAME OIL
Sesame oil is an oil that is extracted from sesame seeds and is most often used in cooking as a seasoning, but in Ayurveda, it is also used for massage and skin care. It has been used for thousands of years in India due to its healing effects.

In Ayurveda, regular massage with sesame oil is recommended to achieve many health benefits. Ayurveda practitioners believe that massage with sesame oil cleanses; balances the lymphatic system and the endocrine system; lubricates; and softens muscles, tissues and joints. They also believe that the oil makes the skin radiant and youthful. Sesame oil is the best oil to use due to its ability to penetrate the skin and because it is generally recommended for all body constitutions, whether you are a vata, kapha or pitta.

According to Ayurveda, sesame oil is excellent because it is naturally antibacterial against common skin pathogens, such as staphylococci and streptococci, and common skin fungi, such as athlete's foot. It is also naturally antiviral and anti-inflammatory.

Additionally, sesame oil is considered to relieve or cure psoriasis, dry scalp, irritated skin, and skin rashes in teens, regulate pore enlargement; and heal or protect wounds.

AYURVEDIC MASSAGE IN THE HOME

How to do Ayurvedic oil massage at home.

1. Before starting the massage, warm the oil to body temperature or higher. Start by massaging your head. Dip your fingertips into the oil and massage the oil into the scalp. During the entire massage, use as much of the entire palm of your hand as possible, not just the fingertips. Since the head is one of the most important body parts to massage, feel free to spend a little more time there than for the other parts.

2. Gently lubricate the face and outer ears. Massage with the entire palm where possible. Massage your face and neck gently. Do not massage as strongly here as on other body parts.

3. Then go on to the neck and upper spine. Massage with open hands and light movements.

4. It is good if you first apply the oil on all body parts and then start again from the top and massage. In this way, the oil has time to stay on the skin for a longer time.

5. Continue with your arms. Massage with reciprocating movements (long up and down movements) along the long muscles and with circulating movements over the joints.

6. Proceed to the chest and abdomen. Massage over the heart with light circular motions. Massage the abdomen clockwise from the lower right side, upwards, to the lower left side.

7. Massage all parts of the back and spine as far as you can.

8. Continue with the legs. Massage with reciprocating movements along the large muscles and with circulating movements over the joints.

9. Finally, massage your feet. Just like the head, the feet are considered one of the most important body parts to massage. Feel free to spend a little more time here. Massage the soles of the feet with the entire palm.

10. Finish with a hot bath or shower.

LESSON NO. 7

LONG SHAVASANA – DEAD MAN'S POSTURE/RELAXATION.

SUPTA PAWANMUKTASANA – THE LEG LOCK.

SHAVASANA – DEAD MAN'S POSTURE.

SURYA NAMASKARA – SUN SALUTATION WITHOUT BREATHING.

SHAVASANA – DEAD MAN'S POSTURE.

PASCHIMOTTANASANA – THE PLIERS.

MATSYASANA – THE FISH.

SHAVASANA – DEAD MAN'S POSTURE.

SHAVA UDARAKARSHANASANA – THE UNIVERSAL POSITION.

SHAVASANA – DEAD MAN'S POSTURE.

SARPASANA – THE SNAKE.

SHASHANKASANA – THE HARE.

SHAVASANA – DEAD MAN'S POSTURE.

YOGA NIDRA – DEEP RELAXATION.

KAYA STHAIRYAM & AJAPA JAPA – STEP 1 + 2 + 3 + 4 – MEDITATION.

END WITH – HARI OM TAT SAT, 3 TIMES.

THEN – OM SRI DURGAYAI NAMAH, 1 TIME.

INSTRUCTIONS FOR ASANAS LESSON NO. 7

LONG SHAVASANA – DEAD MAN'S POSTURE /RELAXATION.

Execution: See module 1.

SUPTA PAWANMUKTASANA – THE LEG LOCK.

Execution: See module no. 1 & 2.

SHAVASANA – DEAD MAN'S POSTURE.

Execution: See module no. 1 & 2.

SURYA NAMASKARA – SUN SALUTATION WITHOUT BREATHING.

Execution: See module 3.

SHAVASANA – DEAD MAN'S POSTURE POSTURE.

Execution: See module no. 1 & 2.

PASCHIMOTTANASANA - THE PLIERS.

Execution: See module 2.

MATSYASANA – THE FISH.

Execution: See module 2.

SHAVASANA – DEAD MAN'S POSTURE.

Execution: See module no. 1 & 2.

SHAVA UDARAKARSHANASANA – THE UNIVERSAL POSITION.

Execution: See module 1 & 2.

SHAVASANA – DEAD MAN'S POSTURE.

Execution: See module no. 1 & 2.

BHUJANGASANA – THE COBRA.

Execution: See module 2.

SHASHANKASANA – THE HARE.

Execution: See module 1 & 2.

SHAVASANA – DEAD MAN'S POSTURE.

Execution: See module no. 1 & 2.

YOGA NIDRA – RELAXATION.

Execution: See module 3.

KAYA STHAIRYAM & AJAPA JAPA – STEP 1 + 2 + 3 + 4 – MEDITATION.

Execution: See module 3.

BINDU VISARGA (READ ABOUT THE CHAKRANA IN MODULE 4)

To practice regularly for a month.

Moorcha pranayama. Sit in a meditation position. Practice kechari mudra. Inhale - slowly and deeply, through both nostrils with ujjayi pranayama while tilting your head back and performing shambhavi mudra. Experience the Bindu. Keep your arms straight by pressing your hands against your knees. Then bend your arms while slowly exhaling with ujjayi and pointing your head forward and closing your eyes. Then relax completely and experience a sensation of lightness and calm in the body. About 10 rounds or more.

Vajroli / sahajoli mudra with concentration on Bindu. Sit in a meditation position. Squeeze the urethra without activating the ashwini mudra or moola bandha. Pinch for 10 seconds, and relax for 10 seconds. Continue like this for about 5 minutes. Every time you pinch, you experience Swadhisthana chakra at the tailbone and say – Swadhisthana, 3 times. Then go via sushumna up to Bindu and say – Bindu, 3 times. Then return to Swadhisthana and relax. Up to 25 rounds. NOTE. In this context, this exercise should be practiced directly after the moorcha pranayama as these together activate and locate the Bindu visarga.

The experience of the inner sound. Practice the bumblebee first – bhramari pranayama, for a while. 5-10 minutes. Put your index fingers in your ears, close your eyes and hum quietly to yourself. Then sit in the same sitting position with your index fingers in your ears and be completely silent. Listen for the first best sound in your head. Then isolate this sound. You use this sound to increase your consciousness. Just experience this sound – nothing else. After a while, you can hear an even more subtle sound in the background – then you concentrate on this sound and gradually use the same technique to penetrate more deeply into the subtle vibrations of the head. 10 minutes or more.

Shanmukhi mudra. Sitt i siddhasana / siddha yoni asana. Sit on a pillow that touches the Mooladhara chakra. Relax. Then use your fingers to close your ears (thumb), eyes (index finger), nose (middle finger), and mouth (ring & little fingers). Then release the pressure against the nostrils - inhale, close again with your fingers and hold your breath. Listen to sounds from the Bindu, the middle of the head or the ears. Then go from the rough sounds to the fine ones. Do not stop for too long at a sound. 5-10 minutes. Shanmukhi mudra means – to close the 7 openings (to the outer world and start listening to the inner – mind).

KNOWLEDGE TEST MODULE 7

ANSWER AS FULLY AS YOU CAN, THEN CHECK IF YOU ANSWERED CORRECTLY. PRACTICE UNTIL YOU KNOW THE ANSWERS BY HEART.

1. EXPLAIN WHAT AYURVEDA IS.

2. DESCRIBE THE DOSHAS.

3. EXPLAIN ABOUT THE YOGI AND AYURVEDIC DIET.

4. DESCRIBE THE SIX TASTES.

5. DESCRIBE THE ASANAS FOR VATA.

6. DESCRIBE THE ASANAS FOR PITTA.

7. DESCRIBE THE ASANAS FOR KAPHA.

8. EXPLAIN WHAT PULSE DIAGNOSTICS ARE.

9. WHAT IS BINDU VISARGA?

10. DESCRIBE SOME POWERFUL EXERCISES TO EXPERIENCE BINDU VISARGA.

MODULE 8

**ESOTERIC YOGA. WE ARE STUDYING SOME OF THE MOST ADVAN-
CED YOGIC TECHNIQUES TO AWAKEN THE DORMANT POWER
WITHIN US**

*We study some of the most advanced techniques for awakening Kundalini Shakti
within us and become acquainted with the tantra of the right and left paths. We
read about secret chakras, magical mantras, Kriya yoga as well as maithuna and
sex magic. We study the Sahasrara chakra and practice exercises for an integrated chakra awakening. We continue to practice in the role of yoga teacher with
lesson no. 8 of 8.*

*Knowledge test: Answer the questions related to module 8. Practice lesson no. 8
with at least 1 participant and humbly accept feedback from them. Ask questions afterward – how was the pace, did you keep to time, did you speak loudly
enough, and how well did you understand the exercises?*

ESOTERIC YOGA

THE WAY OF HIDDEN KNOWLEDGE

Esoteric means "inaccessible" or "only for the initiated", and is most often used to denote the hidden wisdom or secret spiritual knowledge that underlies philosophical systems. The term esoteric can also refer to the teachings and practices of supersensible experiences that require special preparation and training, often under the guidance of an experienced teacher.

Why is knowledge hidden, one might wonder? The answer is multifaceted, but in addition to the fact that the mysterious and hidden have an appeal to new students, it has a purely practical explanation. For example, if someone is only temporarily curious, they will most likely forget a mantra told to them, even if the mantra could be life-saving. Tradition – the knowledge of it – will go nowhere. If, on the other hand, a person were to undergo demanding yogic and tantric training for years, that person will be more likely to remember the mantra. By keeping the knowledge hidden, it ensures that the knowledge is passed on and preserved for the future.

According to an old prophecy, the hidden, esoteric, tantric acts would one day be practiced quite openly – during Kali's age – which is now. It allows me to write about the most advanced tantric rituals that have previously been hidden. However, I can not reveal everything. I can not tell you everything about things that can be abused. For example, I will not reveal the most powerful mantra there is, the shodasi mantra. A mantra that can replace all other secret mantras and gives the holder the power to influence everything in the macro and microcosm: the power of life and death; success and defeat. However, I can tell you about other previously hidden ones, the rituals that are refined through training and that give the adept an increased awareness and increased vitality to deal with everything in life successfully. There is no point in not telling about that knowledge, in not passing it on. It would be like not telling interested people where they can find the best running shoes. Everything that can make it easier for people to have increased vitality and joy in life must now be acknowledged. The time has come. The time is now. The time is yours. Good luck!

THE PATH OF THE RIGHT AND LEFT HANDS

In tantra – which is the basis of all yoga, the hidden knowledge is preserved in two different directions, or paths. We talk about the path of the right hand (dakshinachara), and the path of the left hand (vamachara). Both paths aim to awaken Kundalini Shakti and give the practitioner cosmic power. The difference is that instead of striving to become one with the divine as in dakshinachara, in vamachara tantra one strives to become divine. However, both paths are considered equal ways of enlightening the Indian tantric practitioners, although vamachara is considered the faster and more dangerous way.

DAKSHINACHARA

Dakshinachara is also described as the inner way or the path of inner meditation. Rituals are based on the practitioner's interior, such as Kriya yoga.

VAMACHARA

Vamachara, the path of external meditation, is often the path that people know in tantra, where the adept gets help from things and experiences in the outside world to expand power. For example, the use of meat and wine in the maithuna ritual (tantric intercourse).

Both paths use secret mantras and yantras in their tantric rituals to achieve their purposes.

MANTRA SHASTRA

Mantra shastra is the foundation of all spiritual practice and has a central role in all esoteric yoga.

MANTRA

The most basic mantra is Aum, also known as the pranava mantra, the source of all mantras.

Two types of mantras which have a literal meaning are:

1.) SAGUNA MANTRA

Mantras that represent and invoke a deity, god or goddess for spiritual self-realization. Saguna mantras create visual patterns through repeated chanting until the deity appears in true form.

Some examples of saguna mantras are:

a) Om Namah Shivaya. Greetings to Shiva.

b) Om Nam Narayanaya. Greeting to God over harmony and balance.

c) Gayatri mantra. Dedicated to the goddess Gayatri.

d) Mahamrityunjaya mantra. Dedicated to Shiva.

More similar mantras are shanti mantra, Ram, Sita, Om Aing Saraswati Namaha, etc.

2.) NIRGUNA MANTRA

Mantras that are formless, abstract and represent the universe as a whole and not in any specific form are called nirguna mantras. These mantras require a higher form of concentration as they do not refer to any actual form. They are for deeper meditation and with regular practice, siddhis (paranormal abilities) are obtained.

The use of nirguna mantras is primarily to become one with the absolute or to identify with the divine in the universe.

Some examples of nirguna mantras are:

a) Om (Aum).
Om is the original mantra, the root of all sounds and letters that create language and thoughts.
b) So Ham.

We unconsciously utter this mantra every time we breathe. On inhalation – So, and on exhalation – Ham. So Ham means – I am that, beyond the limitations of the mind and body, I am one with the infinite. I am. That's me.

There are primarily ten different types of magic mantras without a literal meaning:

1. Shanti (Siddhi) mantra – to free oneself from disease, fear, imagination and other problems.
2. Stambhan mantra – to make living beings unable to move.
3. Mohana mantra – used to create attraction.
4. Uchchatan mantra – used to create mental imbalance in people.
5. Vashikaran mantra – used to turn someone into a slave.
6. Akarshan mantra – used to acquire wealth and material happiness.
7. Jrambhan mantra – used to change human behavior.
8. Vidweshan mantra – used to make two people enemies.
9. Maran mantra – used to kill someone.
10. Paustik mantra – used to become a successful person on all levels.

SRI VIDYA MANTRA – SHODASI MANTRA

Sri yantra – also known as Sri Chakra – is called the mother of all yantras because all other yantras are descended from it. It is the most powerful yantra and symbolizes the creation of the cosmos and all life. Sri Vidya is worshiped by the tantric of both the right and left hands.

SRI YANTRA

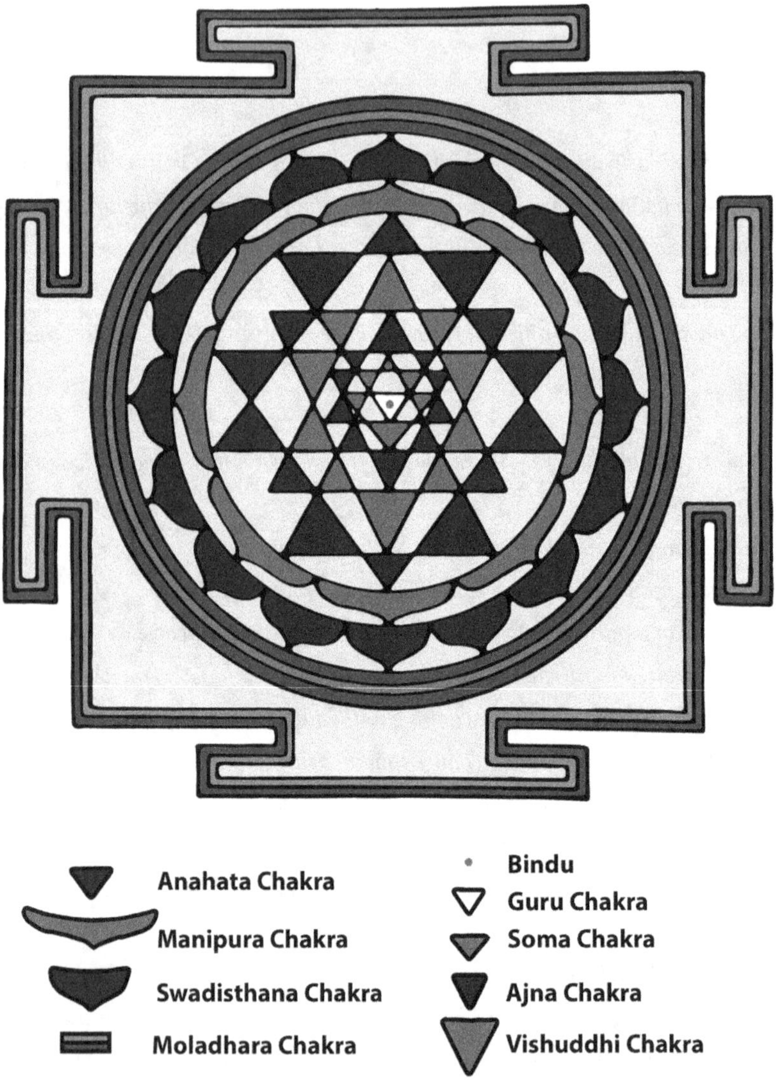

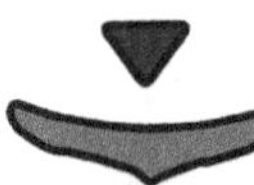 Anahata Chakra

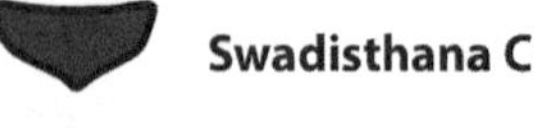 Manipura Chakra

Swadisthana Chakra

Moladhara Chakra

Bindu

Guru Chakra

Soma Chakra

Ajna Chakra

Vishuddhi Chakra

Sri Vidya or Sri Chakra represents Sri Lalita or Tripura Sundari – Shakti in her most beautiful form, a sixteen-year-old beauty. Sri Lalita is represented by sixteen syllables as she is also associated with sixteen desires.

Since Sri yantra is the most powerful yantra, it also possesses the most powerful mantra – the shodasi mantra. It is quite logical if you think about it, as each form also has a sound.

The shodasi mantra is the most secret and protected mantra there is and is completely impossible to find out about – unless you are initiated by a guru. Forget all the pages on the internet that claim to know the mantra because it is completely wrong and unreasonable. If you have undergone all the trials that it means to be initiated, you just do not give it away – especially not on the internet.

Normally, one does not initiate the shodasi mantra directly; it is the guru who decides which time and place is most favorable. Generally, you are first initiated in the bala mantra, then depending on your maturity and insight, you are initiated in the panchadasi mantra. The panchadasi mantra is a mantra made up of fifteen stages syllables. If the guru then thinks that the adept is ready for final liberation, he is initiated into the shodasi mantra and gains knowledge of the secret sixteenth stage.

For the adept to achieve complete liberation and obtain magical abilities, so-called siddhis, he must recite the mantra nine hundred thousand times and add purascharana each time at the end.

BRAHMA VIDYA – THE BIGGEST SECRET

Shodashi vidya is also referred to as Brahma vidya: Brahman (the world soul) and Vidya (the knowledge). Brahman is rendered into mantra form in shodasi vidya and because of this, it is guarded as the greatest secret.

If the practitioner has the opportunity to reach the fourth level of consciousness, known as turiya (superconsciousness), then it is most likely he is also prepared to go beyond this, to reach the fifth level of consciousness known as turiyatita. Turiyatita can be reached without difficulty when the shodasi mantra is recited regularly.

Therefore, by reaching turiyatita (the fifth level of consciousness) and by reciting the shodasi mantra, you become one with Brahman. There is nothing after this.

What happens when a person is transformed into turiyatita? The soul is replaced by the world soul, the divine consciousness. You become divine and gain divine power.

This is also something that can be experienced in a moment of near death, a person is never the same after such an experience.

BIJA MANTRA

Mantras often used in tantra are bija mantras. They are different sounds that have no direct literal meaning, but that have the power to create a great transformation and expansion of the physical, emotional and mental forces. They are called bees or seed mantras, or so-called magical sounds.

The approximately fifty sacred sounds from the Sanskrit alphabet (bija mantras) are primarily resonants for the seven major chakras. Properly stated, they activate the energy in different chakras and purify and balance the mind and body. They also increase the power of various mantra compositions.

AIM

After Om (Aum) the second most common bija mantra is Aim, pronounced – Aym. The Aim is the feminine aspect of Om and often follows Om in various mantras. Om and Aim consist of two compound vowels and therefore include all sounds. A + u creates Om and A + i creates Aim.

Om helps to purify the mind and Aim helps to focus in different ways.

Just as Om is the sound of the invisible, Aim is the sound of the visible. Om is the sound of the unmanifested and Aim is the sound of the manifested. The principle of consciousness and energy. Shiva and Shakti. Therefore, one can often hear Aim in Shakti mantras. Mantras of the Divine Mother.

The Aim is the bija mantra for Saraswati, the goddess of knowledge and speech. Aim helps us in education, art, expression, and communication and is good for all forms of school work in general. The Aim is also a guru mantra and helps us to have greater knowledge of everything. It also helps us with concentration during the recitation of the mantras.

HRIM

After Om and Aim, Hrim, pronounced "Hreem", is the most common bija mantra. It is a combination of the sound Ha, which stands for energy/prana, space and light with the sound of Ra, which stands for fire, light and learning; and the sound A, which stands for energy, concentration and motivation.

Hrim is bija mantra for Shakti or Parvati.

Hrim is a mantra for magic, attraction, love and power. It brings us joy, ecstasy, passion, and complete happiness.

Hrim is a specific mantra for the heart (hridaya in Sanskrit) on all its different levels: spiritually, emotionally, as a chakra, and as a physical organ.

SRIM

Srim, pronounced "Shreem", is one of the most common bija mantras due to its positive properties. It attracts everything that is good, favorable and helps us develop positively.

Srim is the bija mantra of Lakshmi, and is also called the Ramas bija, when used for the worship of Lord Rama.

Srim is the mantra of faith, devotion, refuge and surrender. It can be used to take refuge in or indulge in various deities and obtain their favors.

Srim relates to the heart more from a feminine and sentimental perspective, while Hrim relates to the heart from a masculine, pranic or functional perspective.

Srim is often used with Hrim as Hrim relates to the sun and Srim relates to the moon.

KRIM

Krim is pronounced "Kreem", and is the most important bija mantra that begins with a harsh consonant. Krim begins with Ka, the first consonant in Sanskrit and which shows manifested prana and the initial phase of energy. To Ka, it adds the Ra sound – the sound of fire and the A sound that concentrates power like the other Shakti mantras. Krim creates light just like Hrim and Srim but on a more specific and actualized level.

Krim is the bija mantra of Kali, the goddess of time, destruction and transformation. Kali also creates the highest energy level within us.

Krim is the mantra of work, yoga and the energy of transformation. It is known to be a bija mantra for yoga practitioners and is applied to awaken Kundalini Shakti within us. Krim stimulates higher perceptiveness and higher prana and works to stabilize pratyahara within us. The mantra can create contact with any deity.

KLIM

Klim is pronounced "Kleem" and is the softer, more feminine aspect of Krim. Just as Krim is electric, Klim has a magnetic quality and attracts things to us.

Klim relates to Akarshana Shakti or the law of attraction. Klim is the bija mantra for Krishna and Sundari, the goddesses of love and beauty. It is also the bija mantra over all desires (kama bija) and helps us achieve our inner desires in life. Klim is the mantra of love and devotion and increases the level of love within us. Because of this, it is one of the most used mantras.

STRIM

Strim, pronounced "Streem", is composed of the Sa sound which stands for stability and the Ta sound which creates expansion, with the A sound which provides us with energy, direction and motivation.

Strim is known to be the peace mantra, the so-called shanti bija. The mantra Strim provides the power to have children, to enrich something nutritionally, to protect and to guide. It is similar to Srim but stronger and has a more stabilizing effect.

Strim is the bija mantra of the Hindu goddess Tara (not the Buddhist Tara). Hindu Tara is associated with Durga, often called Durga-Tara, a guarding and protective form of the goddess.

HUM

Hum is pronounced "Hoom", and is one of the most important bija mantras along with Om, Aim and Hrim. It is said to be Pranava, the sound of Lord Shiva.

Hum is the great agni or fire mantra and can increase the fire within us at all different levels. Everything from the fire of consciousness, the pranic fire, and to the burning of the body.

Hum is also a weapon, a protecting mantra that can be used to destroy negativity with its enlightening fire. It is also called the bija mantra of anger (krodha bija).

Hum relates to a violent form of the goddess, like Kali, Chandi or Chinnamasta. Hum is especially used to raise Kundalini Shakti in combination with breathing and with a concentration on the navel (Manipura chakra).

THE SECRET CHAKRAS

In yoga, people usually talk about seven or eight larger chakras that are located along the spine and at the top of the head. If you count Bindu visarga as a chakra, then you say that there are eight major important chakras in a human being. Bindu is located on the top of the back of the head and, according to popular belief, has no kshetram.

In the hidden tradition, you get to learn a big secret: that Bindu's placement on the back of the head is the chakra's kshetram. That Bindu is located above the Sahasrara chakra and is called Sunya. When the Kundalini Shakti reaches the Sunya – the black chakra, one is transformed into a deity and receives divine qualities.

In addition to Sunya, other chakras are hidden: Guru, Nirvana, Indu, Manas and Tala (Lalana) chakras are placed in the head and Hrit chakra is placed just below the Anahata chakra, the heart chakra.

THE HIDDEN RITUALS

KRIYA YOGA

There are a total of seventy-two kriyas, of which twenty are the most used and are suitable for daily use by any student. These kriyas are divided into three groups:

1. Those who evoke pratyahara.
2. Those who evoke dharana.
3. Those that induce dhyana.

KRIYAS FOR PRATYAHARA:

VIPAREETA KARANI MUDRA

Come into vipareeta karani asana. Make sure that the legs are straight and that the chin does not touch the chest. Close your eyes and breathe ujjayi pranayama. Experience in an inhalation how the amrit or nectar flows along the spine from the Manipura to the Vishuddhi chakra and gathers there. Hold your breath for a while and experience how the nectar gets cool. Then exhale with ujjayi breathing and experience how the nectar flows from Vishuddhi through Ajna, Bindu and Sahasrara. After exhaling, take the consciousness to Manipura again and repeat the kriya a total of twenty-one times.

CHAKRA ANUSANDHANA

Sit in a meditation position and close your eyes. Breathe normally. Take consciousness to the Mooladhara chakra and follow the front passage "arohan" up to the Bindu. Silently repeat all the chakras on the way up Mooladhara, Swadhisthana, Manipura, Anahata, and Vishuddhi and go from here directly to Bindu. Then let the consciousness go down along the back passage and repeat the chakras on the way down. Starting from Ajna, Vishuddhi, Anahata, Manipura, Swadhisthana and finally Mooladhara. Then start immediately on the next round starting with Swadhisthana. Do not overdo it by trying to locate the chakras but flow past them easily. Practice nine rounds.

NADA SANCHALANA

Sit in a meditation position. Exhale completely. Open your eyes and bend your head down without pressing your chin against your chest. Take consciousness to the Mooladhara chakra. Silently repeat "Mooladhara, Mooladhara, Mooladhara". Inhale and let the consciousness flow through the anterior passage "arohan" up to Bindu. Repeat the names of the chakras on the way up. When passing from Vishuddhi to Bindu, tilt your head slightly backward. Hold your breath and say "Bindu, Bindu, Bindu", silently to yourself. Then continue down the back passage "awarohan" while saying the mantra Om inwardly. Close your eyes as you go down and experience the chakras. When you arrive at Mooladhara, hold your breath and repeat "Mooladhara" three times. Then continue directly to the next round. Practice thirteen rounds.

PAWAN SANCHALANA

Sit in a meditation position and close your eyes. Practice khechari mudra and ujjayi pranayama. Exhale completely and tilt your head down as in the previous kriya. Become aware of the Mooladhara chakra and silently repeat "Mooladhara, Mooladhara, Mooladhara". Then inwardly say "arohan" and inhale with ujjayi breathing along the front passage while experiencing the chakras and mentally repeating their names. When you pass from Vishuddhi to Bindu, tilt your head back and silently repeat "Bindu, Bindu, Bindu". Then inwardly say "awarohan" and exhale along the back passage with ujjayi breathing. Repeat the name of the chakras silently and close your eyes slowly as you move down. Then open your eyes, tilt your head down and start the next round. Practice forty-nine rounds.

SHABA SANCHALANA

Sit in a meditation position. Practice khechari mudra and ujjayi pranayama. Exhale completely and open your eyes. Bend your head forward and pay attention to the Mooladhara chakra for a few seconds. Inhale with ujjayi breathing and ascend along the anterior passage. Experience what the sound of breathing So sounds like on the way up. Experience each kshetram at the same time without any mental repetition. Tilt your head back at the transition from Vishuddhi to Bindu. Hold your breath and experience Bindu for a few seconds. Exhale, close your eyes and hear the sound of the breath, Ham. Experience each chakra on the way down without rehearsing mentally. When you get to Mooladhara, open your eyes and bend your head and start the next round. Practice fifty-nine rounds.

MAHA MUDRA

Sit in siddhasana or siddha yoni asana with your heel pressed against the Moo-

ladhara. Practice khechari mudra, exhale completely and tilt your head forward. Keep your eyes open at first. Silently repeat "Mooladhara, Mooladhara, Mooladhara". Climb upwards along the "arohan" with an ujjayi inhalation. Experience each kshetram on the way up. Raise your head as you pass from Vishuddhi to Bindu. At Bindu, repeat "Bindu, Bindu, Bindu", internally. Practice moola bandha and shambhavi mudra while holding your breath. Repeat mentally "shambhavi, kechari, mool". When you say "shambhavi", focus your attention on the eyebrow center. When you say "kechari", focus your attention on the tongue and palate. When you say "mool", focus your attention on the Mooladhara chakra. Repeat this procedure three times, accustomed practitioners repeat it twelve times. The first release the shambhavi mudra and after that the moola bandha. Become aware of Bindu and walk down the back passage with ujjayi breathing to the Mooladhara chakra. Experience each chakra on the way down. With Mooladhara, tilt your head forward and open your eyes. Repeat "Mooladhara, Mooladhara, Mooladhara" and continue to the next round. Practice twelve rounds and finish with "Mooladhara, Mooladhara, Mooladhara".

MAHA BHEDA MUDRA

Sit as in the previous exercise. Practice khechari mudra and exhale completely. Keep your eyes open. Mentally repeat "Mooladhara, Mooladhara, Mooladhara". Inhale with ujjayi and ascend along the anterior passage to Bindu. As you pass from Vishuddhi to Bindu, lift your head. Repeat mentally "Bindu, Bindu, Bindu". Go down the back passage to the Mooladhara with ujjayi breathing and close your eyes. Experience the chakras on the way down. Then practice jalandhara bandha while holding your breath. Practice nasikagra drishti, uddiyana bandha and moola bandha. Mentally repeat "nasikagra, uddiyana, mool" and experience its seats in the body. Repeat the procedure three times as a beginner and twelve times when you are more accustomed. Release nasikagra drishti, moola bandha, uddiyana bandha and jalandhara bandha. Hold your head down and experience Mooladhara. Repeat "Mooladhara, Mooladhara, Mooladhara", mentally. Continue to the next round. Practice twelve rounds.

MANDUKI MUDRA

Sit in bhadrasana. Keep your eyes open. The body surface under the Mooladhara should be in contact with the floor. Place a pillow or blanket under you if necessary. Place your hands on your knees and practice nasikagra drishti. Become aware of the natural breath that flows through your nostrils. On inhalation, respiration flows through both nostrils and meets at the eyebrow center. On exhalation, the flow separates at the eyebrow center and flows out through the nostrils. Experience how the flow of breathing follows a V-shaped pattern. Be aware of all odors. The point of the kriya is to experience the smell of the astral body which is the smell of sandalwood. If your eyes get tired, close them for a while. Do the exercise until it feels intoxicating. Do not get caught in it but quit before you are absorbed by it too much.

TADAN KRIYA

Sit in padmasana with your eyes open. Place your hands next to your body on the floor with your fingers pointing forward. Tilt your head back and practice shambhavi mudra. Inhale through the mouth with ujjayi breathing. When you inhale, experience how the breathing sinks downwards through a tube that goes between the mouth and the Mooladhara chakra. Hold your breath, experience the Mooladhara chakra and practice the moola bandha. Using your hands, lift your body off the floor and lower it so that the Mooladhara lightly hits the floor. Repeat three to eleven times. Then exhale through the nose with ujjayi breathing. Practice seven times.

KRIYAS FOR DHARANA:

NAUMUKI MUDRA

Sit in a meditation position. Keep your eyes closed throughout the exercise. Make sure to have pressure at Mooladhara, use a pillow or blanket if necessary.
Make the khechari mudra and bend your head gently downwards. Mentally repeat "Mooladhara, Mooladhara, Mooladhara". Inhale through the anterior passage to the Bindu. Raise your head as you pass from Vishuddhi to Bindu.

Practice shanmuki mudra. Block the ears with the thumbs, the eyes with the index fingers, the nostrils with the middle fingers, the upper lip with the ring fingers and the lower lip with the little fingers. Practice moola bandha and varjoli/sahajoli mudra. Experience the passage along the spine to Bindu. Visualize a trident in copper at the bottom of the Mooladhara. The shaft runs along the spine and the prongs point upwards from Vishuddhi. The trident rises spontaneously several times and its middle prong pierces Bindu. When it pierces Bindu, you mentally say "Bindu bhedan". After a while, release the varjoli/sahajoli mudra, moola bandha and drop your hands on your knees. Exhale from the Bindu with ujjayi breathing along the posterior passage and down to the Mooladhara. Say "Mooladhara, Mooladhara, Mooladhara", mentally. Repeat the exercise. Practice five rounds and finish by exhaling.

SHAKTI CHALINI

Sit in a meditation position. Keep your eyes closed throughout the exercise. Practice khechari mudra. Exhale completely, tilt your head forward and experience Mooladhara. Mentally repeat "Mooladhara, Mooladhara, Mooladhara", and then ascend along the front passage to Bindu with ujjayi breathing. Lift your head when you reach Bindu. Hold your breath and practice shanmukhi mudra. Let the consciousness flow continuously down the back passage and up along the front passage while holding your breath. Visualize a narrow green snake moving along the psychic passage. Its head is at Bindu and it bites its tail. When you follow the snake, you can see how it starts to move along the passage or even make its passages. Look at the snake no matter what it does. When you need to exhale, release your hands and experience Bindu. Go down the back passage with ujjayi pranayama. Repeat "Mooladhara, Mooladhara, Mooladhara", and ascend again along the front passage. Practice five times without interruption.

SHAMBHAVI

Sit in a meditation position. Close your eyes and practice khechari mudra. Visualize a lotus flower with a long green stalk extending downwards. The roots are white or transparent green. The roots spread outwards from the Mooladhara chakra. The lotus flower is at the Sahasrara chakra and is closed like a bud. At the bottom of the bud are some light green leaves. The fallen petals of the flower are pink with fine red veins. Try to see the lotus. You visualize it in chidakasha and feel it all over your body. Exhale and take consciousness to the root of the Mooladhara chakra. Inhale with ujjayi breathing and let your consciousness rise along the stem that rises upwards along the spine. At the end of inhalation, you reach the bud of the flower. Keep your attention on the Sahasrara and hold your breath. You are inside the lotus flower but you can also see it from the outside. It begins to unfold slowly. When the flower opens, you can see its yellow pollen sprinkled in the middle. The lotus closes and opens almost immediately again. When the lotus has stopped opening and closing, exhale with ujjayi and go down the stem to the Mooladhara. Stay there for a while and experience how the roots spread in different directions. Repeat the exercise eleven times.

AMRIT PAN

Sit in a meditation position. Keep one eye closed and practice khechari mudra. Take consciousness to the Manipura chakra. A warm sweet liquid is stored there. Exhale completely with ujjayi while taking a quantity of fluid to the Vishuddhi chakra along the spine. Stay at Vishuddhi for a while. The liquid that you took with you from Manipura is now cooled down. With ujjayi breathing you exhale up to the Lalana chakra. Inflate the cold fluid up to the Lalana chakra using the breath. Take consciousness to the Manipura chakra again. Repeat the exercise nine times.

CHAKRA BHEDAN

Sit in a meditation position. Keep your eyes closed throughout the exercise. Practice khechari mudra and ujjayi pranayama. Breathe without interruption between inhaling and exhaling. Exhale and take consciousness to the Swadhisthana chakra. Inhale and take consciousness to the Mooladhara chakra and then up along the anterior passage. At Vishuddhi kshetram, breathing will end and you will start exhaling immediately. Exhale from Vishuddhi kshetram to Bindu and then down the spine from Ajna to Swadhisthana chakra. This is a complete round. Practice fifty-nine rounds. If you become too introverted, finish the exercise and move on to the next kriya.

SUSHUMNA DARSHAN

Sit in a meditation position, close your eyes and breathe normally. Take consciousness to the Mooladhara chakra. Imagine a pencil with which you draw a square at the Mooladhara chakra. Draw an inverted triangle inside the square. Then make a circle that touches each corner of the square. Make four petals on each side of the square. Take consciousness to Swadhisthana. Draw a circle there, as big as the previous one. Draw six petals around the circle and a crescent moon inside it. Take consciousness to Manipura. Draw a circle and draw an inverted triangle inside it. In the middle of it, you draw a fireball. Make ten petals around the circle. Take consciousness to the Anahata. Draw two triangles that lie on top of each other, one with the tip up, and the other with the tip down. Draw a circle around these with twelve petals. Then take consciousness to Vishuddhi. Draw a circle with a smaller circle inside like a drop of nectar. Make sixteen petals around the circle. Take consciousness to the eye. Draw a circle with the sign Om inside. Draw two large petals around the circle, one on the right side and one on the left side. For Bindu, draw a crescent moon with a very small circle above it. At Sahasrara, make a circle with a triangle with the tip facing up. There are a thousand petals around the circle. Try to see all the chakras in their respective places. It can be difficult to see everything at once, start by seeing two at a time and add a new one for each day.

PRANA AHUTI

Sit in a meditation position. Close your eyes and breathe normally. Experience a light pressure on the top of the head, the pressure of a divine hand. The hand provides the body and mind with prana flowing down from the Sahasrara along the spine. You may experience this as cold, heat, electricity, or as a stream of liquid or wind. When the prana has reached the Mooladhara chakra, you go directly to the next kriya.

UTTHAN

Sit in a meditation position. Close your eyes and breathe normally. Take consciousness to the Mooladhara chakra. Try to visualize it as detailed as you can. See a black shiva lingam. The bottom of the lingam is cut away and a small red snake moves around it. The snake tries to entangle itself so it can rise up along the sushumna. While it struggles to get rid of it, it makes an angry hissing sound. The tail is attached to the Shiva lingam but the body and head rise up along the spine and then come down again. You may experience this as the body contracting followed by a feeling of happiness and bliss. When this occurs, move on to the next kriya.

SWAROOPA DARSHAN

Sit in a meditation position and keep your eyes closed. Become aware of your physical body. Your body is completely still. You are as solid as a mountain. Become aware of your natural breathing while making sure your body is completely still. Your body solidifies and becomes immobile. After a while, you are absorbed by the natural breath while your body continues to solidify. When your body is so still that you cannot move it even though you want to, you move on to the next kriya.

LINGA SANCHALANA

Sit completely still with your eyes closed. Your breathing has automatically switched to ujjayi breathing and you are practicing khechari mudra. Be fully aware of your breathing. With each inhalation, the body expands and with each exhalation, it contracts. Your physical body is still completely still; it's your astral body that moves. After a while, you only experience the astral body. You may reach a stage where the astral body during contraction becomes a small point of light. When this happens, you go straight to the next kriya.

KRIYA FOR DHYANA:

DHYANA

You have experienced your astral body as a small point of light. Take a closer look at the bright spot and how it takes the shape of a golden egg. When you look at the egg, it begins to expand. As it gets bigger, it starts to get the same shape as your astral and physical body. This form is neither material nor subtle in any way: it is the form of pure light.

MAITHUNA:

PREPARATION

Everything that precedes the act itself is apt to raise awareness and remove tensions.

1. The room where the ritual is to take place is clean, incense should burn there. The nose and the olfactory organs are connected by nerves and fine psychic currents to the Mooladhara chakra, where the Kundalini is twisted. When the sense of smell is properly affected, your attention and sensitivity increase.

2. Prepare food and flowers to be used during the ritual. The meal consists of four different parts and the room is decorated with flowers.

Pancha makara, tattwa chakra or pancha tattwa is also the name of the five "m" used in the ritual.

Wine – madya.

Wine symbolizes the intoxicating experience of the richness of consciousness, achieved through yoga. If you prefer not to use alcohol, you can replace it with non-alcoholic wine or coconut milk. The element fire. Tattwa agni.

Meat – mamsa.

Flesh symbolizes, "Everything I am, everything I do and experience – what I stand for, everything is part of my being." If you do not eat meat, replace it with garlic, ginger, sesame seeds, tofu or other soy products. The element earth. Tattwa prithvi.

Fish – matsya.

Fish symbolizes a state where "I experience everything, the whole universe, pleasure and pain, as myself. I am all this. I contain all opposites ". If you do not eat fish, replace it with aubergines and radishes. The element water. Tattwa apas.

Roasted barley products – mudra.

Rice, wheat, etc. They symbolize that, "I stop identifying with fears and inhibitions". The element air. Tattwa vayu.

Flowers (represents intercourse) – maithuna.

Flowers symbolize intercourse, which in turn symbolizes the original power, the feminine that rises to the highest chakra and there unites with the masculine. The element space. Tattwa akasha.

3. Shower together. It is relaxing and invigorating and prepares you both to meet your "divine partner". Shakti (the woman who symbolizes all women) is lubricated with fragrant oils and perfumes. Different oils can be rubbed into different parts of the body, such as musk oil around the Venus mountain.

Then you especially massage your partner's spine. Start at the lower part of the spine and press your thumbs alternately with small movements back and forth and work your way up along the spine. The area where the sushumna, ida and pingala nadi flow, is then released from tension and activated.

TO OPEN UP

The room has been decorated with flowers, the food has been served and the wine has been poured, incense glows, candles are burning or even better, an oil lamp that emits a red glow.

The next step in this exalted experience is to inaugurate and cleanse the room and the house by sprinkling water and saying a mantra. A mantra with long lines of verse is usually used.

This part of the ritual is extensive and precisely laid out to keep the mind occupied. The mind comes in an elevated and secure state. Here you can use the mantra – Am Hrim Krom Hamsah So-Ham, which is repeated out loud eleven times. To the house or surroundings, to the room, to those present, to the food, to the wine, to the four directions, up and down. The different bija mantras are often translated as different manifestations of energy and consciousness. In this context, however, the mantra as a whole represents "conscious attention".

Have a small bowl of water in front of you, dip your fingers in it and sprinkle the water as above and say the mantra Swaha (I burn it, I donate it) each time. Also, dip some flowers in the water and throw them on the food – Swaha, on the wine – Swaha, on those present - Swaha ...

This act should last so long and be so thorough that you become completely pre-occupied with it and can indulge in it seriously and without reservation.

With his finger dipped in red powder mixed with a little soapy water and oil, Shakti puts a red dot on the eyebrow center of those present. She also gets a point. This symbolizes the ability for concentration and empathy achieved through the Ajna chakra in the middle of the head. If Ajna's chakra is aroused, you will participate in this act without tension, without being hampered by shame or frivolity.

YOGA AND MEDITATION

Do pranayamas and bandhas and yoga nidra. Then use the mantra So-Ham (or your mantra) with ujjayi pranayama. Meditate for a while with So-Ham – So as you inhale, and Ham as you exhale. So-Ham means "I am that – I am part of the divine, I am God". Meditate on your body. Experience your natural breathing until you reach a deep and calm state, then repeat the mental mantra Am Hrim Krom Hamsah So-Ham. Experience your body as light – imagine that the body is made of pure light and that this light destroys every fear in you, every inhibition and all hatred. Experience that you are prepared for the cosmic act. You experience the union between the power – the feminine in you, and the consciousness – the masculine. Experience a strengthening and cleansing light flow that fills your entire body and your breathing.

RITUALS

If several people are present, a guru is appointed to lead the ritual. He dips his middle finger in the water and draws a downward-pointing triangle on the floor where you sit and then over this he draws an upward-pointing triangle. In the middle of both triangles – in the middle of the hexagonal star, draw a smaller square and in the square another downward-pointing triangle. A circle that touches all the corners is drawn around both triangles, then eight petals are drawn around the outside of the circle.

The two triangles symbolize the female and male parts of the universe. Shiva and Shakti. Purusha and Prakriti. Consciousness and energy. The square symbolizes the foundation from which the power is aroused and rises, the Mooladhara chakra. The force, Kundalini, is symbolized by the last triangle. The circle symbolizes eternity. The petals symbolize infinity.

Finally, before the action itself, an important part of the ritual comes: the wine is inaugurated by Shakti with flowers, water and the mantra Swaha. She opens the wine to everyone present. The wine has a liberating effect on the mind, but do not drink too much. Consciousness must pass clearly.

The man sits in a meditation position. The woman sits on his left thigh. They give each other wine and food, feeding each other. If this position is too difficult, you can sit next to each other with the woman sitting to the left of the man.

Just as scents affect Mooladhara chakra, Swadhisthana chakra is affected by food and drink. All this increases the desire and sensitivity.

THE ACT

Sit opposite your partner – look each other in the eyes. You are completely naked – two people, a man and a woman, and experience each other's sex and desire. You appreciate each other; two divine beings, who participate in a universal action.

Meditate on each other, and experience each other with desire and joy. If you smile from embarrassment or tense muscles in your face or body, return to the relaxed naturalness every time. Get back to the game and the seriousness of what you do, over and over again. If limiting thoughts arise – whatever happens, accept it and then return to the experience of each other.

Continue to experience your divine partner for a long time. You do not have to demand, explain or excuse anything. You should not achieve anything – just be, experience, enjoy!

The intercourse itself can be performed either in the following way or in one of the sixty-four tantric positions. In the tantric positions, you take a sexual yoga position. It is not done mechanically or by you getting up and sitting down again; it is done without you losing touch with each other even for a second. remain immobile in every position...

POSITIONS

1. The man sits in a meditation position and the woman sits down on the man and wraps her legs around the man's waist and hips so that her feet are crossed behind his seat.

2. Same as 1 – but instead of the woman crossing her legs behind him, she lifts them, while the man holds his arms under her knees and embraces her around the waist and lower back.

3. The man is lying on his back and the woman is squatting on him.

4. The woman starts by sitting as in 3, then she lies down backward between the man's legs and stretches her legs along his body.

5. Standing. The man stands on the floor and holds the woman, while she hangs on him with her legs and arms wrapped around him.

6. The woman lies stretched out on top of the man or vice versa. There are several different variations, the back must be straight or by the yoga position. Remain immobile in the position, while you experience each other mentally and physically, together you go into an uninterrupted sexual meditation. You are immobile. The experience of mental and physical union can come at any time and when it comes, stay in it as long as it is at its peak, then end it.
The shortest time in a position is probably a little more than half an hour to reach any real transformation.

However, you do not have to worry about the body or the performance, let the Shakti in your partner lead you and your inspiration. Give and receive. Do not strive for a normal orgasm, but let the experience of each other transform you. The sixty-four different positions symbolize freedom from expectations, so each time you can do things differently. You decide for yourself.

Get used to the ritual, do it many times. Gradually you will master it and get the full benefit of it. When it can be done effortlessly, it will have a deeper effect.

In addition to the ritual performed by a couple, there are rituals shared by several couples sitting together in a circle. The introductory part of the ritual is *performed by all couples together. The woman chosen to be Shakti for all present in the circle symbolizes power and is honored to be one. She pours the wine and leads the serving of the food and thus begins the ritual. A guru performs the mantra ritual and guides the meditation and the process. During intercourse itself, in the different positions, each pair sits separately in a large circle called the chakra. The feast or ritual that raises consciousness is called puja – chakra puja.*

Meditating with others creates a strong force field and provides support to everyone who participates. There are different puja: In the bhairavi chakra you have a partner who is appointed in advance. In yogini puja, you choose freely and independently of the individual.

A chakra puja can be done in different ways. Having intercourse as a ritual is so important that it can have a liberating effect on our lives. It becomes a beautiful and central act in human society.

SEX MAGIC

Sexual power and orgasm create life and are the strongest energy in the cosmos. Therefore, it is used in yoga, tantra and magic to give the practitioner the ultimate power. It is quite logical and easy to understand if you think about it.

After initiating sexual magic, you become a magician. The initiation takes place from man to woman and from woman to man. The guru – regardless of gender, passes on his magical powers to the adept via shaktipat. The adept is initiated with the guru's orgasm.

Even if you do not possess the magical power of a magician, you can use your sexual magic rituals to get what you want, such as magical desire.

MAGICAL WISH

1. Write down / draw your wish on a piece of paper or use a picture of what you wish. Put it next to you and say the wish out loud to yourself.

2. Start masturbating and experience an inner image of desire in the Mooladhara chakra. Experience how the image is in the chakra and turns dark red. Experience four petals that enclose the image.

3. Experience how you draw the image to the Swadhisthana chakra and how the image turns orange in color and how six petals enclose it.

4. Experience how you draw the image to the Manipura chakra and how the image turns yellow and how ten petals enclose it.

5. Experience how you draw the image to the Anahata chakra and how the image turns blue and how twelve petals enclose it.

6. Experience how you draw the image to the Vishuddhi chakra and how the image becomes violet in color and how sixteen petals enclose it.

7. Experience how you draw the image to the Ajna chakra and how the image turns white and how the shape of a pyramid encloses it.

8. Experience how you draw the image to the Sahasrara chakra and how the image turns purple-red and how an infinite number of petals enclose it.

9. When the orgasm comes, you shoot the image out of the Sahasrara chakra and you mentally experience how the desire leaves the scalp and goes away into the cosmos.

Should you change after you have made your magical wish, you will burn up the image of the wish so that it ceases to work.

LESSON NO. 8

LONG SHAVASANA – DEAD MAN'S POSTURE /RELAXATION.

SUPTA PAWANMUKTASANA – THE LEG LOCK.

SHAVASANA – DEAD MAN'S POSTURE.

SURYA NAMASKARA – SUN SALUTATION WITH BREATHING.

SHAVASANA – DEAD MAN'S POSTURE.

VAYU NISHKASANA – THE PUMP.

SHAVASANA – DEAD MAN'S POSTURE.

SHAVA UDARAKARSHANASANA – THE UNIVERSAL POSITION.

SHAVASANA – DEAD MAN'S POSTURE.

BHUJANGASANA – THE COBRA.

SHASHANK ASANA – THE HARE.

SHAVASANA – DEAD MAN'S POSTURE.

YOGA NIDRA – DEEP RELAXATION.

KAYA STHAIRYAM & AJAPA JAPA – STEP 1 + 2 + 3 + 4 – MEDITATION.

END WITH – HARI OM TAT SAT, 3 TIMES.

THEN – OM SRI DURGAYAI NAMAH, 1 TIME.

INSTRUCTIONS FOR ASANAS LESSON NO. 8

LONG SHAVASANA – DEAD MAN POSTURE /RELAXATION.

Execution: See module 1.

SUPTA PAWANMUKTASANA – THE LEG LOCK.

Execution: See module no. 1 & 2.

SHAVASANA – DEAD MAN'S POSTURE .

Execution: See module no. 1 & 2.

SURYA NAMASKARA – SUN SALUTATION WITH BREATHING.

Execution: See module 3. Inhale when opening the body and exhale when folding. For example, inhale into the cobra and exhale into the rock. Hold your breath when lying on your knees, chest and chin.

SHAVASANA – DEAD MAN'S POSTURE.

Execution: See module no. 1 & 2.

VAYU NISHKASANA – THE PUMP.

Execution: See module 3.

SHAVASANA – DEAD MAN'S POSTURE.

Execution: See module no. 1 & 2.

SHAVA UDARAKARSHANASANA – THE UNIVERSAL POSITION.

Execution: See modules 1 & 2.

SHAVASANA – DEAD MAN'S POSTURE.

Execution: See module no. 1 & 2.

BHUJANGASANA – THE COBRA.

Execution: See module 2.

SHASHANKASANA – THE HARE.

Execution: See modules 1 & 2.

SHAVASANA – DEAD MAN'S POSTURE.

Execution: See module no. 1 & 2.

YOGA NIDRA – DEEP RELAXATION.

Execution: See module 3.

KAYA STHAIRYAM & AJAPA JAPA – STEP 1 + 2 + 3 + 4 – MEDITATION.

Execution: See module 3.

INTEGRATED CHAKRA AWAKENING (READ ABOUT THE CHAKRA-NAS IN MODUL 4)

To practice regularly for a month.

Bija mantra sanchalana. Sit in a meditation position and go from the Mooladhara chakra to the Sahasrara chakra with your awareness. At each chakra, you pronounce its Bija mantra and experience how the chakra vibrates in step with the mantra.

Yoga nidra with chakras. Practice yoga nidra and go from Mooladhara chakra to Sahasrara chakra with your awareness. Experience each chakra with its yantra, color, number of petals and bija mantra. Then go down from Sahasrara chakra to Mooladhara chakra and repeat the experience in reverse order.

Image chakras. Draw each chakra as carefully as you can with all its attributes and colors.

KNOWLEDGE TEST MODULE 8

ANSWER AS FULLY AS YOU CAN, THEN CHECK IF YOU ANSWERED CORRECTLY. PRACTICE UNTIL YOU KNOW THE ANSWERS BY HEART.

1. WHAT IS ESOTERIC YOGA?

2. DESCRIBE THE MANTRA SHASTRA.

3. DESCRIBE SHODASI MANTRA.

4. EXPLAIN WHAT THE MANTRA IS.

5. WHAT ARE THE SECRET CHAKRAS?

6. WHAT IS KRIYA YOGA?

7. WHAT IS MAITHUNA?

8. EXPLAIN WHAT SEX MAGIC IS.

9. DESCRIBE THE SAHASRARA CHAKRA.

10. DESCRIBE INTEGRATED CHAKRA AWAKENING EXERCISES.

www.ingramcontent.com/pod-product-compliance
Lightning Source LLC
LaVergne TN
LVHW010314200726
843507LV00010B/1227